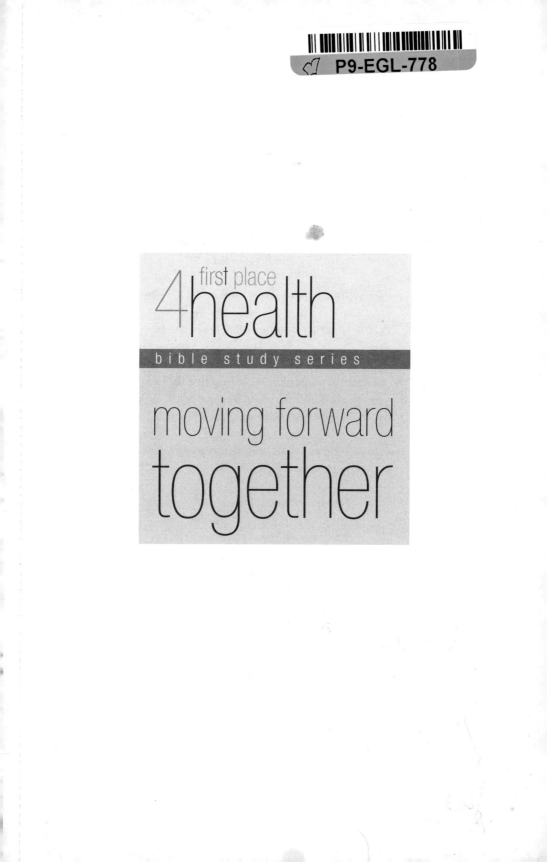

first place
4health
bible study series

moving forward
together

Published by Gospel Light
Ventura, California, U.S.A.
*www.gospellight.com*
Printed in the U.S.A.

**Caution:** The information contained in this book is intended to be solely for
informational and educational purposes. It is assumed that the First Place 4 Health
participant will consult a medical or health professional before beginning this or
any other weight-loss or physical fitness program.

First Place 4 health Bible study.
p. cm.
#2.— Moving forward together
ISBN 978-0-8307-4520-3 (trade paper)
1. Bible—Study and teaching. 2. Christian life—Study and teaching.
I. Title: First Place for health Bible study.
BS600.3.F573 2008
242'.5—dc22
2008006856

Rights for publishing this book outside the U.S.A. or in non-English languages
are administered by Gospel Light Worldwide, an international not-for-profit
ministry. For additional information, please visit www.glww.org, email
info@glww.org, or write to Gospel Light Worldwide, 1957 Eastman Avenue,
Ventura, CA 93003, U.S.A.

# contents

# foreword

My introduction to Bible study came when I joined First Place in March 1981. I had been attending church since I was a small child, but the extent of my study of the Bible had been reading my Sunday School quarterly on Saturday night. On Sunday morning, I would listen to my Sunday School teacher as she taught God's Word to me. During the worship service, I would listen to our pastor as he taught God's Word to me. Frankly, digging out the truths of the Bible for myself had never entered my mind.

Perhaps you are right where I was back in 1981. If so, you are in for a blessing you never dreamed possible. As you start studying the truths of the Bible for yourself through the First Place 4 Health Bible studies, you will see God begin to open your understanding of His Word.

Almost every First Place 4 Health member I have talked with about the program says, "The weight loss is wonderful, but the most important thing I have received from my association with First Place 4 Health is learning to study God's Word." The First Place 4 Health Bible studies are designed to be done on a daily basis. As you work through each day's study (which will take 15 to 20 minutes to complete), you will be discovering the deep truths of God's Word. A part of each week's study will also include a Bible memory verse for the week.

There are many in-depth Bible studies on the market. The First Place 4 Health Bible studies are not designed for the purpose of in-depth study, but are designed to be used in conjunction with the rest of the program to bring balance into your life. Our desire is for each member to begin having a personal quiet time with God each day. This time alone with God should include a time of prayer, Bible reading and Bible study. Having a quiet time is a daily discipline that will bring the rich rewards of balance, which is something we all need.

God bless you as you begin this exciting journey toward a balanced life. God will richly bless your efforts to give Him first place in your life. Remember Matthew 6:33: "But seek first his kingdom and his righteousness, and all these things will be given to you as well."

*Carole Lewis*
First Place 4 Health National Director

# introduction

First Place 4 Health is a Christ-centered health program that emphasizes balance in the physical, mental, emotional and spiritual areas of life. The First Place 4 Health program is meant to be a daily process. As we learn to keep Christ first in our lives, we will find that He is the One who satisfies our hunger and our every need.

This Bible study is designed to be used in conjunction with the First Place 4 Health program but can be beneficial for anyone interested in obtaining a balanced lifestyle. The Bible study has been created in a five-day format, with the last two days reserved for reflection on the material studied. Keep in mind that the ultimate goal of studying the Bible is not only for knowledge but also for application and a changed life. Don't feel anxious if you can't seem to find the *correct* answer. Many times, the Word will speak differently to different people, depending on where they are in their walk with God and the season of life they are experiencing. Be prepared to discuss with your fellow First Place 4 Health members what you learned that week through your study.

There are some additional components included with this study that will be helpful as you pursue the goal of giving Christ first place in every area of your life:

- **Group Prayer Request Form:** This form is at the end of each week's study. You can use this to record any special requests that might be given in class.

- **Leader Discussion Guide:** This discussion guide is provided to help the First Place 4 Health leader guide a group through this Bible study. It includes ideas for facilitating a First Place 4 Health class discussion for each week of the Bible study.

- **Two Weeks of Menu Plans with Recipes:** There are 14 days of meals, and all are interchangeable. Each day totals 1,400 to 1,500 calories and includes snacks. Instructions are given for those who need more calories. An accompanying grocery list includes items that will be needed for each week of meals.

- **First Place 4 Health Member Survey:** Fill this out and bring it to your first meeting. This information will help your leader know your interests and talents.

- **Personal Weight and Measurement Record:** Use this form to keep a record of your weight loss. Record any loss or gain on the chart after the weigh-in at each week's meeting.

- **Weekly Prayer Partner Forms:** Fill out this form before class and place it into a basket during the class meeting. After class, you will draw out a prayer request form, and this will be your prayer partner for the week. Try to call or email the person sometime before the next class meeting to encourage that person.

- **Live It Trackers:** Your Live It Tracker is to be completed at home and turned in to your leader at your weekly First Place 4 Health meeting. The Tracker is designed to help you practice mindfulness and stay accountable with regard to your eating and exercise habits. Step-by-step instructions for how to use the Live It Tracker are provided in the *Member's Guide.*

- **Let's Count Our Miles!** A worthy goal we encourage is for you to complete 100 miles of exercise during your 12 weeks in First Place 4 Health. There are many activities listed on pages 249-250 that count toward your goal of 100 miles. When you complete a mile of activity, mark off the box listed on the Hundred Mile Club chart located on the inside of the back cover.

- **Scripture Memory Cards:** These cards have been designed so that you can use them while exercising. It is suggested that you punch a hole in the upper left corner and place the cards on a ring. You may want to take the cards in the car or to work so that you can practice each week's Scripture memory verse throughout the day.

- **Scripture Memory CD:** All 10 Scripture memory verses have been put to music at an exercise tempo in the CD at the back of this study. Use this CD when exercising or even when you are just driving in your car. The words of Scripture are often easier to memorize when accompanied by music.

Use each of these important tools found in this study to live a balanced and healthy life.

# welcome to
# *Moving Forward Together*

At your first group meeting for this session of First Place 4 Health, you will meet your fellow members, get an overview of your materials and find out what you can expect at weekly meetings. The majority of your class time will be spent learning about the four-sided person concept, the Live It Food Plan, and how change begins from the inside out. You will also have a chance to ask any questions about how to get the most out of First Place 4 Health. If possible, complete the Member Survey on page 201 before your first group meeting. The information you give will help your leader tailor the next 12 weeks to the needs of the whole group.

Each weekly meeting begins with a weigh-in for members. This will allow you to track your progress over the 12-week session. Your Week One weigh-in/measurement will establish a baseline of comparison so that you can set healthy goals for this session. If you are apprehensive about weighing in every week, talk with your group leader about your concerns. He or she will have some options for you to consider that will make the weigh-in activity encouraging rather than stressful.

The day after your first meeting, begin Week Two of this Bible study. This session, you and your group will explore the importance of pressing on toward the goal of healthy balance in every area of your life, and the value of encouraging each other along the way. Instead of falling prey to discouragement and doubt, your path can grow brighter every day—when you and your fellow First Place 4 Health members allow God's Word to show you the way! As you open yourself to the truth of Scripture and share your hopes and struggles with the members of your group during the next 12 weeks, you'll find yourself becoming the healthy child of God you are designed to be!

## Week Two

# step
# by step

Scripture Memory Verse
*I press on toward the goal to win the prize for which*
*God has called me heavenward in Christ Jesus.*
Philippians 3:14

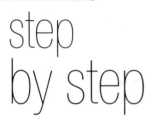

Starting the journey toward health and wholeness through the First Place 4 Health program is easy. In the beginning, we are full of energy and enthusiasm. Visions of a new body fill our mind as we anticipate success. "This time will be different," we tell ourselves and those beginning this journey with us. "This time I will not let other things throw me off course and keep me from realizing my health and fitness goals."

During the first week of each new First Place 4 Health session, we diligently plan our meals, make time for exercise, read Scripture and pray for God's help and guidance. But all too soon the fateful day arrives when our motivation and enthusiasm begin to wane. Other commitments start to press in on us, and obligations like work and family and friends wage war against this new commitment we have made to loving self-care. Before long, we are driving though the fast-food lane again rather than cooking a healthy meal. The morning comes when we skip our daily exercise time, vowing that we will resume it tomorrow— a tomorrow that somehow turns into a week of tomorrows. Our Bible begins to collect dust on the shelf beside the favorite chair we don't have time to sit in. Our prayers are rushed and demanding, not pleasant time spent in communion with God.

Yes, the beginning is easy; but all too soon, life on the world's terms—the instant-results, rapid-paced society we call our world—quickly takes its toll. Weeks later, we look at our shattered health and fitness dreams and wonder what went wrong. Our intentions had been so good, the program had offered so much promise, and we were so sure that this time would be different. But in the end, what began so well turned out to be an instant replay of past failures.

If this scenario sounds all too familiar to you, take heart! This time *can* be different. This session of First Place 4 Health can be the beginning of a bright new future. The present doesn't have to be an instant replay of the past. The Bible says that "the end of a matter is better than its beginning" when we are willing to do things according to God's prescribed plan (Ecclesiastes 7:8). Instead of falling prey to discouragement and doubt, our path can grow brighter every day—when we allow God's Word to show us the way. Victory in Christ Jesus can be ours—we can press on toward the prize for which God has called us heavenward in Jesus!

## PRESS ON   Day 1

*O Lord, as I press on toward my health and fitness goals, help me to replace my impatience with persistent effort that produces lasting results. Amen.*

Our memory verse for Week Two of the *Moving Forward Together* Bible study begins with a bold three-word statement:

I _____ on.

In order to fully understand what Paul is saying in the rest of the sentence, we must first correctly comprehend the meaning of the word "press." Look up the verb "press" in a dictionary, and write the meaning you feel most accurately expresses what Paul meant by the word "press" in our memory verse.

_____

_____

The first definition given in the *Webster's New World College Dictionary* reads, "To act with steady force or weight; push steadily against; squeeze."[1] How is this meaning different from the scenario described in the introduction of this week's Bible study?

_____

_____

_____

How can you apply the words "steady force" to your First Place 4 Health program so that you will not lose motivation as the days and weeks go by? (The key to this answer is contained in the words "win the prize" from this week's memory verse.)

How is a lifestyle characterized by fitness and health different from going on a quick-fix diet?

The second part of the definition listed above for the word "press" is "push steadily against," which implies resistance. What type of resistance might you encounter as you begin this session of First Place 4 Health? All of us encounter many forms of resistance, so list as many as come to mind.

How are the words "push steadily against" similar to the words "steady force" found in the first part of the definition?

The third part of the definition above for the word "press" is "squeeze." Most of us who struggle against the battle of the bulge are very familiar with the word "squeeze," especially as it applies to squeezing into clothing that has become too tight. But obviously that isn't what Paul is talking about in this verse. How can the word "squeeze" be applied to your First Place 4 Health program in a beneficial way?

*Gracious God, I do want the end of my health and fitness efforts to be better than the beginning. Please send Your Holy Spirit to guide me into all truth as I begin to press on toward the prize You have for me in the First Place 4 Health program. Amen.*

## EYES ON THE PRIZE

*Loving Father, help me to always keep the prize You have for me in the First Place 4 Health program foremost in my mind so that I will not grow weary and lose heart. Amen.*

During yesterday's lesson, we looked at the various meanings of the word "press" as it applies to the phrase "press on" from this week's memory verse. What did you learn yesterday that will help the end be better than the beginning during this session of First Place 4 Health?

Our memory verse does not advocate that we press steadily forward just because we enjoy exerting ourselves! We are called to press on for a specific purpose. What is that purpose, according to this week's memory verse?

Because First Place 4 Health is a health and fitness program that emphasizes balance, it is important that we define what the prize we are pressing on toward looks like. All too often we concentrate on physical appearance rather than the inner qualities that give us the ability to press on in the face of obstacles. As we begin this session of First Place 4 Health, list the goals you have for yourself for this leg of your health and fitness journey.

Physically: _____

_____

Mentally: _____

_____

Emotionally: _____

_____

Spiritually: _____

_____

What will happen to your ability to press on if you neglect any of these essential elements of your being? (In answering this question you might want to push against a physical object with both hands, applying more pressure with one hand than the other, to see what happens.)

_____

_____

_____

If you were to push according to the different levels of strength you have in each area of your life, would your efforts to press on result in a straight path, or would you veer to one side or the other, and why?

_____

_____

_____

Which of the four aspects of your being is weakest, which is strongest and which two are in between? Rate your ability to press on in each of the four areas by listing them from strength (1) to weakness (4).

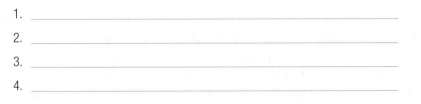

1. _____
2. _____
3. _____
4. _____

After doing this exercise, what steps can you take to shore up your weakest area by relying on your strength so that you can press on with steady effort?

_____

_____

_____

In the introduction to this week's Bible study, we looked at the first portion of Ecclesiastes 7:8. Turn to this passage in your Bible and read the entire verse. What is better than pride?

How is pride like boasting about success in First Place 4 Health but failing to apply steady effort over time?

The key to having the end turn out better than the beginning, according to Ecclesiastes 7:8, is what?

How is patience part of pressing on toward the prize, and how is patience like applying steady effort in a balanced way? Explain your answer thoroughly.

## THE ONE WHO CALLS US HEAVENWARD

**Day 3**

*O Lord God, it is so easy for me to imagine that I am in charge, when in fact I can't do any good thing aside from Your sustaining power and love. Amen.*

Our Scripture memory verse for the week gives us another valuable piece of information about this journey we are making toward health and fitness. Who does Paul tell us has called him heavenward?

Now turn to John 15:16. What does Jesus tell His disciples in this verse?

_____

_____

_____

How does this statement correspond with what Paul says in this week's memory verse?

_____

_____

_____

How does knowing that God is the One who has called you to participate in First Place 4 Health give you the motivation to apply consistent, steady pressure to your First Place 4 Health program?

_____

_____

_____

According to John 15:16, Jesus told His disciples to bear _____ —not just any type of fruit, but fruit that will _____ . How is bearing fruit that will last part of the patient, persistent effort implied in the words "press on"?

_____

_____

_____

What is "fruit that will last" as it applies to the First Place 4 Health program? Make your answer relevant to the four aspects of your being.

Physical fruit that will last:_____

_____

_____

Mental fruit that will last: _____

_____

_____

Emotional fruit that will last: _____

_____

_____

Spiritual fruit that will last: _____

_____

_____

How does this list compare with the goals you made in these four areas during yesterday's lesson, and why?

Physically: _____

_____

Mentally: _____

_____

Emotionally: _____

_____

Spiritually: _____

_____

Can we produce fruit that will last in the four aspects of our being without steady effort over time? Why or why not? (You might want to read James 5:7-8 as you think about your answer.)

_____

_____

_____

How is the production of fruit that will last different from the quick-fix, instant-results diet and exercise programs touted by the world?

_____

_____

_____

In our memory verse, Paul tells us that God has called him _____ .
What is the difference between being called heavenward and being in heaven
with God?

_____

_____

_____

What can this difference teach us about the importance of pressing on with
steady, consistent, patient effort rather than settling for the quick-fix schemes
offered by the world?

_____

_____

_____

*Thank You, loving Lord, that You have called me heavenward. I realize that being called
heavenward implies that I am on a lifelong journey, not an instant-transformation
track. Help me to be patient with the process. Amen.*

Day
4

## IN GOD'S GRIP

*My Lord and my God, my goal is to know You better and to live a life
pleasing to You. Amen.*

In order to really understand all that this week's memory verse has to teach
us, we not only need to correctly comprehend the meaning of the words the
apostle Paul used, but we must also look at the verse in the context of Paul's
entire letter to the Philippians. Turn to Philippians 3 in your Bible, and read
verses 10-16.

According to Philippians 3:10-11, what is Paul's primary motivation?

_____

_____

_____

How does this motivation compare to the goals you set for yourself in First Place 4 Health?

How is doing a daily Bible study in connection with your First Place 4 Health program part of knowing Christ and learning about the power of His resurrection?

Paul was a very mature Christian when he wrote the letter to the Philippians, but had he already been made perfect (verse 12)?

What does this tell you about this heavenward journey we are on during our present life?

Paul first uses the words "press on" in Philippians 3:12. According to this verse, what is Paul pressing on to take hold of?

How does the fact that Paul is pressing on to take hold of that for which Christ had taken hold of him further explain the statement in our memory verse about pressing on toward the prize for which God has called him heavenward?

Pause for a moment and apply Paul's words in Philippians 3:12 to your First Place 4 Health program. What similarities do you find in your First Place 4 Health journey and Paul's words?

_____

_____

_____

Paul says he has not yet been made perfect. Can we expect to be made perfect this side of heaven? Explain your answer.

_____

_____

_____

How is knowing more about Jesus Christ part of the heavenward journey we are making through the First Place 4 Health program? (You will need to ponder all Paul is saying in Philippians 3:10-16 in giving this answer.)

_____

_____

_____

In Philippians 3:16, what does Paul admonish us to do?

_____

_____

What have you attained thus far in the First Place 4 Health program that you need to live up to?

_____

_____

_____

Are you living up to the calling you have received in Christ Jesus? First identify the calling as it applies to health and fitness, and then describe how you are or aren't living up to that call.

_____

_____

_____

*O Father, forgive me for those times when I know what to do but don't do it! Amen.*

## CONSIDER THE COST

*O Lord, You do not ask that I impetuously rush into discipleship but that I carefully consider the cost before making a commitment to follow You. Amen.*

According to this week's memory verse, what does Paul say we must do to win the prize for which God has called us heavenward?

---

What new information have you learned about pressing on during this week's Bible study lessons?

---

There is one more thing we need to consider as we set out on our journey. Turn to Luke 14:25-33. Summarize what Jesus said in your own words.

---

According to Luke 14:28, what did Jesus say we should do before we begin a project?

---

Have you sat down and estimated the cost of being in the First Place 4 Health program to see if this is a cost you can—and will—pay? In answering this question, please do not think in terms of money; think in terms of the time, energy and effort it will take to press on toward the prize! What might First Place 4 Health participation cost you? Make your answer specific to the four aspects of your being.

Physical cost: _____

_____

_____

Mental cost: _____

_____

_____

Emotional cost: _____

_____

_____

Spiritual cost: _____

_____

_____

Are you willing to pay these costs? Why or why not?

_____

_____

_____

According to 2 Samuel 24:24, David made a statement about offering a sacrifice to the Lord. What did David say?

_____

_____

_____

How do David's words help you better understand the true cost (not just the financial price) of First Place 4 Health?

_____

_____

_____

Luke 14:29-30 talks about what will happen to the person who does not carefully consider the cost. What is the result of poor planning?

_____

_____

_____

_____

Recall a time when you began a diet and exercise program without first carefully considering the cost. What was the result when you could not finish what you began?

_____

_____

_____

_____

What was the hidden cost of that program—what kept you from finishing what you had started?

_____

_____

_____

_____

How does careful planning help ensure success, especially when it comes to pressing on toward the prize?

_____

_____

_____

_____

_Thank You, gracious God, for inviting me to consider the true cost of First Place 4 Health so that I will not look foolish when I start a project I am unable to bring to completion. Amen._

Day
6

## REFLECTION AND APPLICATION

*Thank You, Lord, that I can always begin with the end in mind as
I consider the course set before me. I will strive to take hold of
that for which Christ Jesus has taken hold of me. Amen.*

Although we like to think of our life journey toward health and fitness as a straight, level path, for most of us this journey more closely resembles a series of switchbacks going up the side of a steep mountain. We set our goals and begin the climb, but at times this winding passage is difficult to follow. We are always in danger of losing our direction and footing, perhaps taking a shortcut that promises to be the easy way but in the end leads nowhere. As our memory verse for Week Two reminds us, the first thing we need to do is fix our eyes on the prize that awaits us at the end of the journey. And once we have gotten a clear vision of our goal, we then press on toward that goal with patient, persistent effort. Another thing that can help us as we set out toward our destination is to begin with the end in mind and then work our way backward to our starting point.

For a practical example of this principle, get a maze-type puzzle from a book or magazine. Instead of starting at the entrance and finding your way through the network of dead ends until you get to the exit, do it backward. Begin at the exit and trace the route in reverse, until you reach the entrance point. For some reason it's easier that way, both when working a maze puzzle on paper and when getting to our health and fitness goals. When we focus on the desired outcome and figure out what we need to do to get there, we are less likely to get caught in the maze.

Using the trace-your-path-backward technique, identify one action you need to take today in each area of your being to move forward toward your First Place 4 Health success. You identified your goals in our Day Two study, so use those as your starting points and trace them backward to identify the actions you need to take.

Physical: _____

_____

_____

Mental: _____

_____

_____

Emotional: _____

_____

_____

Spiritual: _____

_____

_____

Having identified one step you can take in each area today, challenge yourself to take the steps you have outlined as you press on toward the prize!

*Thank You, Lord, for sending the Holy Spirit to guide me and direct my course as I navigate this maze called life. Amen.*

## REFLECTION AND APPLICATION

Day
7

*O Lord, I can only overcome the forces that keep me in doubt and despair because Jesus overcame the power of sin and death for me. Amen.*

This week we carefully examined our Scripture memory verse so that through deeper understanding of the words, we can better apply the truths of God's Word to our First Place 4 Health program. As you reflect on this week's memory verse, think about what you have learned during this week's study.

There are three little words at the end of our memory verse that we did not talk about. What are those three words?

_____

As we conclude this week's study, take a moment to examine your relationship to Jesus Christ. Have you claimed Him as your Savior and Lord? Has Christ taken hold of you as part of God's eternal plan to give you eternal life through belief in His Son and the price He paid for your redemption? Describe your relationship with Jesus.

_____

_____

Read the words of Romans 8:16. If the Spirit is not confirming in your heart that you are a child of God, please spend time in prayer, asking Jesus to come into your heart and be the Lord of your life. If you have doubts about your eternal salvation, talk to your pastor, your First Place 4 Health leader or a mature Christian friend to help you understand the importance of confessing Christ and allowing Him to be your Lord and your Savior. But even before you have an opportunity to talk to someone about your faith in Jesus Christ, you can accept Him as your Savior in the stillness of your own heart by praying the following prayer. If you made a profession of faith years ago, perhaps you would like to use the prayer to reaffirm your belief that Jesus is Lord:

> *Gracious and loving Father, I humbly confess that I have broken Your laws and my sins have separated me from You. I am truly sorry, and I want to turn away from my past sinful life so that I can turn toward You. Please forgive me, and help me avoid sinning again. I believe that Your Son, Jesus Christ, died for my sins, was resurrected from the dead, is alive and hears my prayer. I invite Jesus to become the Lord of my life, to rule and reign in my heart from this day forward. Please send Your Holy Spirit to help me hear Your voice and obey Your commands. It is my desire to do Your will and bring honor and glory to You in all I say and do. In Jesus' name I pray. Amen.*

Having accepted Jesus as your Lord, be sure to follow through and contact someone who can help you publicly affirm the truth you have stated in your heart. Until Jesus, "the way and the truth and the life" (John 14:6), is your personal Lord and Savior, you will not be able to press on toward the prize for which God has called you heavenward in Christ Jesus, so please don't delay. We're moving forward together and want you to be part of the company of saints moving toward health and fitness on our heavenward journey in Christ Jesus our Lord.

> *Thank You, Jesus, that You are standing at the door of my heart, knocking and asking to come in and have fellowship with me. Amen* (Revelation 3:20).

**NOTE**

1. *Webster's New World College Dictionary,* 3rd ed., s.v. "press."

## *Group Prayer Requests*

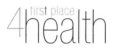

Today's Date: _____

| Name | Request |
|------|---------|
|      |         |
|      |         |
|      |         |
|      |         |
|      |         |
|      |         |
|      |         |
|      |         |
|      |         |
|      |         |

## Results

_____

_____

_____

_____

_____

_____

_____

*Week Three*

# stepping forward
# in faith

*By faith Abraham, when called to go to a place he would later receive
as his inheritance, obeyed and went, even though
he did not know where he was going.*

HEBREWS 11:8

During the Day Two portion of last week's Bible study, you were asked to list the goals you have for yourself during this session of First Place 4 Health. Review your work, and again list your goals.

Physically: _____

_____

Mentally: _____

_____

Emotionally: _____

_____

Spiritually: _____

_____

Even as we write out the words that comprise our goals in these four important areas of our being, we write them knowing that although we have the language skills to describe what we envision, we have not yet experienced what it will be like when we arrive at these goals. We don't know what it will be like to have a clear, self-disciplined mind that is not filled with obsessive thoughts—especially obsessive thoughts about food. We don't know what it is like to have balanced emotions that do not ricochet out of control and fuel a binge-eating episode. We don't know what it is like to have an intimate, interactive relationship with God—a relationship that is not marred by our out-of-control eating. And we certainly don't know what our physical body will look like when we achieve our health and fitness goals. Yes, we pick a number on the scale, but we do so not knowing if that is the right number—and not knowing what we will look like when we finally get there.

Abraham, the father of our faith, faced the same challenge. What was Abraham's situation, according to our memory verse?

_____

_____

_____

This week we will look at Abraham's pilgrimage to see what wisdom we can glean as we, too, begin our journey of faith into uncharted territory.

## BY FAITH    Day 1

*O Lord God, I know it is impossible to please You without faith.*
*I do believe in You, Lord; please help my unbelief. Amen* (Mark 9:24).

Our memory verse for the week begins with two little words that describe how Abraham began his journey into an unknown land. What are those words?

_____    _____

Earlier in chapter 11 of the book of Hebrews, the unknown author gives us a description of faith. Turn to Hebrews 11:1. What do you learn about faith from this verse?

_____

_____

_____

Who was commended for this type of faith, according to Hebrews 11:2?

_____

_____

Hebrews 11:3 tells us about one of the many results of our faith. What does this verse tell us we understand by faith?

After giving us two examples of ancients who were commended for their faith, the writer of Hebrews gives us another fact about faith. What does Hebrews 11:6 tell us is impossible to do without faith?

What two things must we believe when we come to God in faith, according to Hebrews 11:6?

How is your participation in the First Place 4 Health program a manifestation of your faith that God exists and that He rewards those who earnestly seek Him?

Explain in your own words what it means to "earnestly seek" God and how that might relate to pressing on toward the prize.

*Thank You, compassionate Father, for the assurance that You will reward me when I earnestly seek You. Amen.*

# CALLED AND ACCOUNTABLE

*O Lord God, please help me to hear Your voice and obey Your words
as I move forward toward the wonderful new life You have for me. Amen.*

As we begin today's study, write this week's memory verse.

_____

_____

_____

Yesterday we learned what the words "by faith" mean. Today we will look at what Abraham was called to do. In order to learn about Abraham's call, we must go to Genesis 12:1-5. Notice as you read these verses that Abraham's name is different in this passage. We will learn about Abram's name change later in this week's study.

What was God's specific request of Abram (verse 1)?

_____

_____

According to Genesis 12:1, who would show Abram the land he was being asked to travel toward?

_____

_____

_____

How can this truth also describe your First Place 4 Health journey as you too set out on the trek to an unknown land?

_____

_____

_____

What did Abram have to do before he could begin on his journey to this unknown place?

_____

_____

_____

What might you need to leave behind to receive the future God has in store for you through the First Place 4 Health program? List two specific things you must discard before you can begin the journey to health and fitness.

_____

_____

Genesis 12:2-3 lists the benefits Abram would receive if he was willing to step out in faith. Describe in your own words the benefits God promised to Abram.

_____

_____

How does our memory verse for this week describe the place that Abram would later receive?

_____

_____

Does the word "inheritance" imply that Abram would have to work for the land he was to receive, or does "inheritance" imply that it would be a gift—a blessing God would give Abram? Explain your answer.

_____

_____

_____

What does Genesis 12:4 tell us?

_____

_____

Go back to Genesis 12:1, and read God's call to Abram very carefully. Then read Genesis 12:4-5. Although Abram left as the Lord told him, he did not completely obey God's command. What did Abram do that was contrary to what God asked of him?

_____

_____

_____

Later, Abram's nephew Lot would prove to be a great hindrance to Abram. (You can read about that in Genesis 13–14, if you want to see the result of Abram's disobedience.) What might you be trying to bring along on your journey that will hinder your progress?

_____

_____

_____

What does the last part of Genesis 12:5 tell us?

_____

_____

Even though Abram arrived in Canaan, his journey with God was far from over. What does this tell you about this segment of your First Place 4 Health journey?

_____

_____

*Thank You, Father, that all Your promises are "Yes" and "Amen." You do exactly as You have promised when we are willing to step forward in faith. Amen.*

## BELIEVING GOD

### Day 3

*O Lord, it is so much easier to doubt than to believe that Your words to me are true, especially when my finite mind cannot comprehend Your good, pleasing and perfect plan for my life. Amen* (Romans 12:2).

Our memory verse for the week tells us that Abraham obeyed and went, even though _____ _____ _____ _____
_____ _____ _____ .

If someone were writing a brief description of your First Place 4 Health journey, could that writer say the same thing of you? Why or why not? Don't use generalities; give specific examples of your faith in action—or lack of the same.

_____

_____

_____

Even though Abram obeyed and left as God commanded, there was one part of God's promise that continued to puzzle Abram. Go back and reread Genesis 12:2 to learn what God promised Abram. God promised to make Abram a great _____ . But there was a problem, a problem that was a stumbling block to Abram's faith. Read Genesis 15:1-3 and write down what the problem was.

_____

_____

_____

_____

What was God's reply to Abram's questioning? (See Genesis 15:4-5.)

_____

_____

After God spoke to Abram, what did Abram do, and what was the result? (Read Genesis 15:6.)

_____

_____

_____

God has made a promise to you, too—a promise of health, balance and restoration. Yet there are some pieces missing from the health, balance and restoration equation that cause you to doubt that wholeness is possible. What are the missing pieces that need to fall into place for you as you move forward in First Place 4 Health?

_____

_____

_____

Abram took his questions and complaints to God. Have you done the same? If not, spend some time in prayer, telling God about your dilemma and asking for His help.

_____

_____

_____

Turn to Jeremiah 29:11. According to this verse, what is God's promise to you?

_____

_____

_____

Do you choose to believe God and continue on in faith that His plans for you in the First Place 4 Health program are good, even though you may not completely understand them? Why or why not?

_____

_____

_____

*O Lord, today I will choose to believe that Your plans for me are good, even though I don't understand how You will bring them to pass. Amen.*

## A NEW NAME  Day 4

*O Lord, help me to obey You and continue to walk with you, even when I am filled with doubts and fears. Amen.*

Up until now, we have been learning about the life of Abram. Summarize what you have learned about Abram during the first three days of this week's study.

_____

_____

_____

How does Abram's life parallel your journey to health and wholeness through First Place 4 Health? In giving your answer, don't forget Abram's mistakes—and your mistakes, too!

_____

_____

_____

Abram continued to walk with God even though he did not understand God's plan, and he obediently moved forward even as he had many questions and doubts. God continued to prove Himself faithful to Abram, in spite of Abram's doubts and mistakes. How is this like your First Place 4 Health journey? List some of your questions and doubts, and then describe God's faithfulness to you in spite of your failings.

_____

_____

_____

As the years passed, Abram's hope of having a son continued to dwindle. When Abram was 99 years old, the Lord appeared to him again. Genesis 17:1-2 records the beginning of that conversation. What did the Lord say to Abram that day?

_____

_____

_____

When God appeared to Abram, what did Abram do? (Genesis 17:3 has the answer.) Explain in your own words what it means to "fall facedown" when you are in God's presence. Is this a physical posture or an inner attitude, or both?

_____

_____

_____

In response to Abram's reverence, God continued to speak to him. What does Genesis 17:3-8 tell us that God promised Abram? Restate this passage in your own words.

_____

_____

_____

What happened to Abram's name?

_____

_____

_____

Why did God give Abraham a new name?

God's promises to Abram are called a covenant, or an agreement. Genesis 17:9-10 tells us that Abram had a responsibility under that covenant, too. What was Abraham's responsibility (and that of the descendants he did not yet have)?

Not only did Abraham get a new name, his wife, Sarai, got a new name, too. What did God promise to do for Sarai and what was the new name God gave her? (Read Genesis 17:15-16.)

What did Abraham do when he heard God's words about Sarah? (Read Genesis 17:17.)

Recall a time when you laughed to yourself when you read God's promises and plans for you. What did it feel like when you laughed at God's words? Record your thoughts here or, better yet, in your spiritual journal, confessing to God your amusement and lack of faith.

*O Lord, please forgive me for the times I read Your Word and laugh to myself because I don't believe Your promises to me will ever come true. Amen.*

## RICH REWARDS

*Sovereign Lord, it is so easy for me to forget that Your power can accomplish all that You plan and promise. Help me to recall that power when I am tempted to doubt Your Word. Amen.*

This week we have been reading about the covenant God made with Abraham, promises that from a human standpoint seemed impossible. But then one day the Lord appeared to Abraham again. Turn to Genesis 18:1-15 in your Bible, and carefully read this story. Although the passage tells us that the Lord appeared to Abraham, how many men did Abraham see when he looked up, and what did Abraham do when he saw the men approaching his tent (verses 2-8)?

Although Abraham was the one running here and there to accommodate the visitors, who did the visitors inquire about (verse 9)?

When Abraham told the visitors that Sarah was in the tent, what did the Lord say (verse 10)?

When Sarah, sitting in the tent, heard the Lord's words, what did she do (verse 12) and why?

The first sentence of Genesis 18:14 contains a very precious truth. What is that truth? What do Abraham's and Sarah's ages teach us about starting over in the First Place 4 Health program, regardless of our age?

_____

_____

_____

Years of faith in the face of seeming failure paid rich rewards. Turn to Genesis 21:1-2 in your Bible, and stand in awe of God's power as you read the words contained in these verses. How does the story of Abraham and Sarah confirm that nothing is too hard for the Lord?

_____

_____

_____

What about you? What seems too hard—maybe downright impossible—for you right now when it comes to achieving your health and fitness goals? How can the words "Is anything too hard for the Lord?" help you move forward in faith?

_____

_____

_____

## REFLECTION AND APPLICATION

### Day 6

*O Lord God, so many of the names I have called myself in the past have not supported my profession of faith. Help me, gracious God, to accept the new name You have for me. Amen.*

During our Day Four study, we read about the new names Abram and Sarai received as they stepped forward in faith, not knowing where they were going but trusting in God's words and promises. What new names did God give Abram and Sarai?

_____

_____

_____

One of the sad consequences of carrying too much weight are the names people call us because of our physical size. And this degradation is not limited to the names *others* call us—often our "self-talk" is more harmful than the cruelest words spoken to us by others. Stop for a moment and list the names our society gives people who are carrying excess body fat, and be sure to include the negative names you have called yourself, too.

_____

_____

_____

_____

But praise God! He will also give us a new name, a new identity, as we step forward in faith through participation in the First Place 4 Health program! Now list the names others will give you when you have the body, mind, heart and spirit God has in store for you as you walk obediently with Him. After you've written out this list of new names, circle the two that are your favorites.

_____

_____

_____

_____

What is keeping you from calling yourself those new names right now? Remember, God changed Abraham's name long before Isaac was born, and you can begin calling yourself by a new name long before you reach your destination, too!

_____

_____

_____

_____

*Thank You, Father God, that You give me a new name and a new identity in Christ Jesus my Lord. Amen.*

## REFLECTION AND APPLICATION

*O Lord God Almighty, today I will recall Your goodness to me and give*
*You the worship and praise You deserve. Amen.*

After God first appeared to Abram with a promise of an inheritance Abram would later receive, Abram stepped forward in faith. After he arrived in Canaan, Genesis 12:7 tells us that Abram built an altar to the Lord. Today we are going to build an altar to God to express our thankfulness for God's faithfulness and love. On a separate piece of paper, draw the outlines of 12 large stones arranged in the shape of an altar. (You can use construction paper, but regular copy paper will work just fine, too.) Remember, these are rough, natural stones piled on top of each other, not neatly arranged. Make each of the stones large enough so that you can write a word or two inside each one.

When you have finished constructing your altar, inside each rock write a word or two that tells a way God has been loving and faithful to you through the First Place 4 Health program. You will be sharing your altar at your next First Place 4 Health meeting, so be sure to complete this project and then bring it to your next meeting. Be as creative with this exercise as you like. Those who are very visual or artistic might like to cut the stones in their altar from colored paper and glue them onto another sheet.

*O Lord, You are loving and You are faithful. Thank You for this opportunity to express my thanks and praise for the good things You have done for me. Amen.*

## *Group Prayer Requests*

4 first place
health

Today's Date: _____

| Name | Request |
|------|---------|
|      |         |
|      |         |
|      |         |
|      |         |
|      |         |
|      |         |
|      |         |
|      |         |
|      |         |
|      |         |

## Results

_____

_____

_____

_____

_____

_____

*Week Four*

# receptive to the Word

SCRIPTURE MEMORY VERSE

*But the worries of this life, the deceitfulness of wealth and*
*the desires for other things come in and choke the word, making it unfruitful.*

MARK 4:19

There is a big difference between pressing on toward the prize and having the things of this world press in and keep us from moving forward. During our Week Two lessons, we learned what it means to "press on." Summarize what you learned about the words "press on" during Week Two.

_____

_____

_____

_____

What feelings and emotions are stirred in you when you see yourself pressing on toward the prize that awaits you in the First Place 4 Health program? Describe what it feels like to be moving forward together with God as you consistently do the things that please your Lord and Master.

_____

_____

_____

_____

Now consider the words "press in." What feelings and emotions are stirred in you when you hear the words "press in"? Imagine what it feels like to have commitments and obligations pressing in on you and interfering with your plans and goals. Be honest and creative in writing your description.

_____

_____

_____

_____

Jesus was a master storyteller who often explained spiritual truths by using simple illustrations the common people of His day could easily understand. These stories are called *parables* because they compare an earthly situation—something that people can readily comprehend—with a spiritual truth—something more difficult to understand. One such parable, or teaching story, is called the Parable of the Sower; from this parable we will learn some valuable lessons this week about the importance of feeding what is good and weeding out what is not. In preparation for this week's lessons, read Mark 4:1-20. This passage contains both the parable Jesus told the crowd that day by the lake and the explanation the Lord later gave His disciples so that they would understand what He was teaching through this simple story.

## Day 1 — THE GOOD SEED

*Gracious and loving Lord, thank You for explaining spiritual truth by using simple stories that I can understand and take to heart. Amen.*

Although the Parable of the Sower is about a farmer sowing seed, the true meaning of this story had nothing to do with farmers or seeds or crops. According to Mark 4:14, what is this story really about, and who is the farmer Jesus is talking about?

_____

_____

_____

As Jesus scattered the word-of-God seed among the people on the hillside that day, there were four reactions to the Master's message. In the chart on the following page, describe both the situation used in the parable and the explanation Jesus later gave His disciples.

| Situation in the Parable | Explanation Given by Jesus |
| --- | --- |
| Verse 4 | Verse 15 |
| Verses 5 and 6 | Verses 16 and 17 |
| Verse 7 | Verses 18 and 19 |
| Verse 8 | Verse 20 |

*Father, even as I write these words I am reminded of the times when Your Word did not take root in my heart. Forgive me for allowing the things of this world to interfere with my devotion to You. Amen.*

## QUICKLY TAKEN AWAY

Day 2

*O Lord, Your Word is a lamp to my feet and a light to my path. Please give me the grace to receive Your truth and the strength to follow the path You set before me. Amen (Psalm 119:105).*

As you begin today's study, go back and reread Mark 4:1-20, making note of anything the Holy Spirit brings to your awareness that you did not notice when reading these words yesterday.

What specific words did the Spirit impress on your heart and mind through the reading today?

Why do you think you skipped over those words during yesterday's reading?

_____

_____

_____

Refer to the chart you filled in during your Day One lesson, and tell what the first situation was that Jesus used as He told the crowd this parable.

_____

_____

_____

What was the explanation of that situation Jesus later gave His disciples?

_____

_____

_____

How does this explanation help you understand how you might have missed important truths when you first read this parable yesterday?

_____

_____

_____

Jesus told His disciples that the birds that gobbled up the good seed were an illustration of what Satan tries to do to us when we hear the truth of God's Word. How do daily Bible study and memorizing Scripture verses each week keep Satan from snatching away important spiritual truths?

_____

_____

_____

What does Mark 4:4 tell us about the condition of the soil that produced bird seed rather than a rich crop?

_____

_____

_____

The seed fell on the path, a part of the field that was hard and packed down because it was trampled as people and animals walked on it. The path was probably on the perimeter of the field and exposed to the traffic of the world. What parts of your inner being have been trampled by the things of this world so that those parts cannot receive God's good Word?

_____

_____

_____

What are some of the things of this world that impact your life and harden your heart so that God's Word does not find a nesting spot within you?

_____

_____

_____

Jesus said the birds came along and ate up the seed lying on top of the path. What do some of the "birds"—those things that gobble up the Word before it can penetrate into your heart—look like in your life? Remember that the birds here are an illustration of a much deeper spiritual reality.

_____

_____

_____

How might these "birds" be part of the worries of this life that our memory verse talks about?

_____

_____

_____

What is one thing you can do today to soften your heart so that it will readily receive the Word of God?

_____

_____

_____

How is First Place 4 Health part of that softening process?

_O Lord, I will set aside quiet time to study Your Word and pray so that the evil one does not have a chance to snatch away the spiritual truths You desire to teach me. Amen._

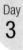

## Day 3

## SHALLOW ROOTS

_O Lord, thank You for inviting me to sit at Your feet and learn from You so that I will be prepared to face the trials that come my way as I strive to move forward with You. Amen._

Yesterday we looked at the first situation regarding our ability to receive the Word of God Jesus described to the crowd and His disciples. What did you learn from yesterday's study?

Refer to the chart you completed during your Day One study and describe the second situation Jesus offered the crowd and the explanation of that illustration He later gave to His disciples.

During the introduction to the Week Two study of _Moving Forward Together_, we looked at the people who begin a new diet and exercise program and are full of excitement, but soon fall away. How are these people like the second illustration Jesus gave in the Parable of the Sower?

What does the Divine Physician diagnose as the cause of the problem that keeps this seed from growing to maturity?

_____

_____

_____

How are daily Bible study, Scripture memory and prayer part of building healthy spiritual roots?

_____

_____

_____

From the second illustration in the Parable of the Sower, what can you learn that reinforces the need to incorporate the mental, emotional and spiritual parts of our being into our physical diet-and-exercise program?

_____

_____

_____

Jesus compared the sun that scorched the young plants to the trouble and persecution that come because of the Word. How have you experienced trouble and persecution that came because you were being obedient to God's Word since beginning the First Place 4 Health program? Give this question careful thought. Much of the trouble and persecution we encounter is very subtle, but it nevertheless erodes our root system.

_____

_____

_____

Does spending daily time in the Word and in prayer help you cope with the trouble and persecution in a way that allows you to flourish rather than wither and fall away? Why or why not?

_____

_____

_____

How are the other members of your First Place 4 Heath group part of the root system that allows you to withstand the trouble and persecution we all encounter when we determine to follow Jesus more closely?

_____

_____

_____

Give a specific example of a time when one of your First Place 4 Health brothers or sisters held you up when you were weak and in danger of withering.

_____

_____

_____

_____

Before you conclude your quiet time, write that person a note of gratitude, telling how he or she has been part of the First Place 4 Health root system that has allowed you to withstand the things that have pressed in on you and threatened to undermine your First Place 4 Health efforts. Spend the remainder of your quiet time thanking God for giving you a healthy root system that can sustain spiritual growth and health.

> *Gracious God, truly You give me everything I need to live a life pleasing to You. I have Your Word, I have Your presence, and I have the people You have given me to be part of the root system that allows me to grow and flourish. Amen.*

## Day 4 — PULLING WEEDS

*Thank You, Father, for sending the Holy Spirit to give me eyes to see, ears to hear and a heart ready to receive Your Word. Amen* (Isaiah 6:10).

As you begin today's study, reread Mark 4:1-20, once again making note of any words the Holy Spirit brings to your attention during the reading. What did you have eyes to see today that was hidden from you in previous readings?

_____

_____

_____

Our Week Four memory verse comes from this passage. Write the memory verse, noting where it appears in Jesus' story. Is it part of the parable or part of the explanation?

_____

_____

_____

How does reading the entire parable and explanation help you better understand what is being taught in this week's memory verse?

_____

_____

_____

Refer to the chart you completed during your Day One study, and in your own words, describe both the third illustration from the parable and the explanation Jesus gave of it to His disciples.

_____

_____

_____

According to this week's memory verse, what are the three specific things that Jesus said keep seed from becoming fruit-bearing plants? Remember, this is not seed the birds gobbled up or seed that sprouted quickly and then withered. This is seed that produced growing plants.

_____

_____

_____

We are in Week Four of our Bible study now, and if you have been faithful to the First Place 4 Health program since beginning this session, the good seed has begun to grow in your heart. You now resemble a plant that has the potential to bear fruit, so Jesus' words have particular application to your continued growth. In the chart on the next page are the three categories of things Jesus warned can press in and choke out the First Place 4 Health program that has taken root and begun to grow in you. Under each category, list at least two things that have the potential to sabotage your progress.

| Worries of This Life | Deceitfulness of Wealth | Desires for Other Things |
|---|---|---|
| | | |
| | | |
| | | |
| | | |
| | | |
| | | |

Now pick one item from each category and describe how you will eradicate that weed before it presses in on you and chokes your ability to press on.

The worry of this life that is pressing in:

_____

_____

_____

How I will press on:

_____

_____

_____

The deceitfulness of wealth that is pressing in:

_____

_____

How I will press on:

_____

_____

The desire for another thing that is pressing in:

_____

_____

How I will press on:

_____

_____

How might a desire for instant results in a diet and exercise program be a worry, a deceit and a desire that has the potential to choke out your First Place 4 Health program? Please give this question careful thought and explain your answer thoroughly.

_____

_____

_____

How can the truth of the First Place 4 Health program be part of your weed-killing arsenal?

_____

_____

*You are so good to me, Lord. When the things of this world press in on me, You give me the strength to press on. Thank You for victory in Jesus. Amen.*

## FAITHFUL AND FRUITFUL

*Sovereign Lord, You call me to be both faithful and fruitful. Help me to press on toward the prize rather than allow the things of this world to press in on me. Amen.*

This week we have been studying the Parable of the Sower, as found in the Gospel of Mark. Summarize what you have learned about the things that keep the good Word seed from becoming fruit-bearing plants.

---

---

---

---

The fourth situation that Jesus described in this parable had an ending much different from the first three situations He told the crowd about that day. Look back at the chart you completed during the Day One study, and tell what the end result of the fourth type of seed is.

---

---

---

What is the explanation Jesus gave His disciples about the fourth situation?

---

---

---

Yesterday we learned that three things kept the growing plants from reaching maturity. What were those three things? (They are from our memory verse for this week.)

---

---

---

According to Mark 4:20, what are the three things that happen to the seed that was sown on good ground?

_____

_____

_____

How is hearing the Word part of your First Place 4 Health program?

_____

_____

_____

What can you do that will allow the Word you hear to sink into your being and produce a good crop? (The answer is found in this week's memory verse.)

_____

_____

_____

But not only do you need to hear the Word, you also need to accept it. How are hearing and accepting two different things?

_____

_____

_____

What part of the First Place 4 Health program have you heard about but not accepted in a way that produces results?

_____

_____

_____

The seed sown on good ground also produces a crop. What type of crop will we produce through faithful participation in First Place 4 Health?

_____

_____

_____

Bearing fruit is about increase, but obviously we are not striving to increase physically through participation in First Place 4 Health! What kind of increase are we working for?

_____

_____

_____

The crop in Jesus' parable varied from plant to plant. Some plants produced 30, some 60 and some even 100 times what was sown. How does this truth speak to our individual differences—and what does it teach us about not comparing our progress with that of others in First Place 4 Health?

_____

_____

_____

The Parable of the Sower also appears in the Gospel of Luke. In his version, Luke gives us a bit of information that is helpful to our First Place 4 Health efforts—and this Bible study. Read Luke 8:15. What other ingredients of faithfulness and fruitfulness do you learn about from Luke's words?

_____

_____

_____

How is persevering akin to pressing on and different from succumbing to those things that press in on us as we move forward together in the First Place 4 Health program?

_____

_____

_____

_____

_____

_O Lord, it is so easy to fall prey to the things of this world rather than persevere long enough to bear fruit. Forgive me for my failings, and give me the strength to press on toward the prize. Amen._

## REFLECTION AND APPLICATION

*Gracious God, it is so easy to read Your Word but not take it into my heart so that it makes a difference in the way I live my life. Forgive me for not applying Your Word to my health and fitness endeavors. Amen.*

Today we are going to revisit the chart we completed on Day One, but this time we are going to add a third column by giving an example of Jesus' parable and explanation as they both apply to First Place 4 Health. Rewrite the words from your Day One study in the first two columns below, and then in the third column, give a First Place 4 Health illustration of the parable's situation.

| Situation in the Parable | Explanation Given by Jesus | First Place 4 Health Illustration |
| --- | --- | --- |
| Verse 4 | Verse 15 | I complete my daily Bible study lessons, but later in the day I can't remember what I read, especially as it applies to out-of-control eating. |
| Verses 5 and 6 | Verses 16 and 17 | |
| Verse 7 | Verses 18 and 19 | |
| Verse 8 | Verse 20 | |

*Lord God, I want to be faithful and fruitful. Help me to hide Your Word in my heart so that I will not sin against You. Amen* (Psalm 119:11).

Day 7

## REFLECTION AND APPLICATION

*Gracious and loving Lord, thank You for the beauty of Your creation and for allowing even the simple things in nature to teach me spiritual truth. Amen.*

As we have seen from the Parable of the Sower, Jesus often used the natural things in God's creation to teach powerful spiritual lessons. Today we are going to go out into the wonderful world God created for our enjoyment to see what lessons the Holy Spirit has for us. You will want to take a bag or tote along to collect the object lessons God brings to your attention during your nature walk. You might also want to take along a pen and paper in case your nature lesson is too large to put in the bag or is something you cannot grasp with your hands (such as clouds). Walk long enough to collect 10 items from nature that reinforce the truths you learned this week as you studied the Parable of the Sower. You will be sharing your findings with your First Place 4 Health group, so be prepared to explain the spiritual truth taught by each of the nature items you chose.

*God of nature and creation, thank You for the beauty of the earth and for giving me the pleasure of walking in Your world. Amen.*

## *Group Prayer Requests*

4health

Today's Date: _____

| Name | Request |
|------|---------|
|  |  |
|  |  |
|  |  |
|  |  |
|  |  |
|  |  |
|  |  |
|  |  |
|  |  |
|  |  |

Results

_____
_____
_____
_____
_____

## Week Five

# over
# it all

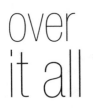

SCRIPTURE MEMORY VERSE
*And over all these virtues put on love,*
*which binds them all together in perfect unity.*
COLOSSIANS 3:14

Those of us with oversized bodies are well versed in what fashion experts call the "layered look." We have spent enormous amounts of money, time and energy learning the art of putting on layer after layer of clothing in an attempt to hide the bulges and ripples we hope to cover up with clothing. As we begin this week's Bible study, stop and think about the lengths you have gone to in an attempt to present the illusion of a slimmer self to the "thin is in" society we live in. Ponder the cost in terms of money, time and energy—at the expense of comfort—that you expended trying to cover an inner problem with fashionable exterior garments. What did your reflection reveal?

---

While most of us do not want to take a closer look at the vices our layers conceal, our Scripture memory verse for Week Five invites us to examine those virtues we are to cover with love. We are to put on some everyday, one-size-fits-all garments before we tie on the servant apron called love, the final piece of spiritual clothing that binds the rest of our virtues together.

## VIRTUES IN VOGUE

*O Lord God, so often I talk about being loving, but when I carefully study Your Word, I quickly learn that I have not put on all the virtues that are the foundation of my spiritual wardrobe. Amen.*

Imagine for a moment that you just received a letter from a dear friend or family member. As you begin to read what you believe to be the second page of that letter, you see the words, "After you have put all these other things together, mix them together carefully and seal them with love." So you quickly look back to page 1 to see what "all these other things" you are to put together consist of. But to your dismay, there is no list. Obviously, there is a page missing in this precious piece of correspondence. That's what we do when we pull our memory verse for Week Five out of context. "Over all these virtues put on love" is an invitation for us to read the verses that precede Colossians 3:14 so that we can discover what these virtues we are to put on look like.

Turn to Colossians 3:12-13 in your Bible, and list the seven virtues Paul tells us to put on before we put on love.

1. _____
2. _____
3. _____
4. _____
5. _____
6. _____
7. _____

What does the word "all" before the word "together" tell us must happen before love can bind the other virtues together in perfect unity (verse 14)?

_____
_____
_____
_____

Carefully look at the list of seven virtues. Which items are missing from your spiritual wardrobe, and what does that tell you about your ability to love God, love yourself and love others?

_____

_____

_____

*Thank You for loving me, Lord, even though I am so prone to put on layers of clothing rather than build a strong, healthy body that I do not need to be ashamed of. Amen.*

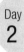

Day
2

## LOVING MYSELF

*O Lord God Almighty, all too often I strive to accommodate others rather than care for my body, mind, heart and spirit as You command. Please forgive me. Amen.*

| Virtue | Loving Self-Care Application |
|---|---|
| Compassion | |
| Kindness | |
| Humility | |
| Gentleness | |
| Patience | |
| Forbearance | |
| Forgiveness | |

Self-care is not something most of us have learned to practice, especially those of us who have a history of abusing our bodies with excess food and little, if any, exercise. Yes, we put on all the virtues Paul lists in Colossians 3:12-13, and when it comes to how we treat others, we do bind them together with love. Yet sadly, how we treat ourselves is a much different matter. Until we allow ourselves to experience the wonder and mystery of God's love and respond by loving God and loving the self He calls precious, we cannot break the cycle that keeps us in despair. The seven virtues that Paul tells us to put on are listed in the chart on the previous page. Next to each virtue, write a brief explanation of how this virtue is part of the loving self-care you are learning to practice through the First Place 4 Health program. As you complete the list, remember these are about how you act toward yourself, not how you act toward others!

Which of these virtues are you most deficient in when it comes to how you treat yourself, and why?

Write this week's memory verse and then underline the word "all."

What can you do today to begin adding the seven virtues from Colossians 3:12-13 to your First Place 4 Health program?

*Mighty and merciful God, You call me to love myself, not because I am perfect, but because I am perfectly loved by You. Thank You for Your goodness and grace. Amen.*

## PUT ON A NEW SELF

*O Lord God, You call me to be a new creation in Christ Jesus. Help me to eliminate the old-self practices that keep me from moving forward in my First Place 4 Health journey. Amen.*

Not only does the apostle Paul tell us about the new virtues we are to put on once our life is rooted and grounded in Christ Jesus, but Paul also tells us what we were like before Jesus saved us. Turn to Colossians 3:5-8 in your Bible, and summarize what Paul says about our former way of life.

_____

_____

_____

Now reflect on the layers we have used to cover up our excess body size. What would we be doing if we tried to cover over the things Paul lists in Colossians 3:5-8 rather than put them to death? (The beginning of Colossians 3:9 has the answer.)

_____

_____

_____

When we attempt to cover up our sins rather than deal with them God's way, who are we are deceiving?

_____

_____

_____

In Colossians 3:9 Paul says, "Do not lie to each other, since you have taken off your old self with its practices." What old-self practices will you need to take off before you can put on the virtues Paul lists in Colossians 3:12-13? Write your answer as a confession to God, who already knows about all the things you need to take off. You might want to use your spiritual journal for privacy.

_____

_____

_____

During yesterday's study, we made a list of the seven virtues Paul lists in Colossians 3:12-13—virtues that are applicable to the First Place 4 Health program. Which of these virtues will you need to put on as you take off the old items that are not part of your new wardrobe in Christ Jesus, and why?

Turn to 1 John 1:8-10. What hope can you glean from these verses—what hope that will allow you to put on the new self that is yours in Christ Jesus?

According to 1 John 1:8, what do we do when we say we are without sin, and how is that like covering up rather than confessing our faults and failings?

One of the virtues we are to put on is humility. How is humility part of admitting we are sinners in need of God's grace?

Why is humility a necessary ingredient for those who are moving forward with God on this journey to health, balance and wholeness? Consider all you have learned during this week's study as you formulate your answer.

Can you accomplish any of the other things on Paul's list of virtues (Colossians 3:12-13) until you have first humbled yourself and admitted your human weaknesses? Why or why not?

_____

_____

_____

*O sovereign Lord, it is so difficult to admit I am human; but until I can confess my sins to You, I cannot put on the new garments You have for me. Amen.*

Day
4

## HUMILITY PAVES THE WAY FOR FORGIVENESS

*O Lord, I am blessed because You have taken away the guilt of my sin. Amen.*

Although God extends His forgiveness to us long before we confess our sins to Him, confession is a necessary part of forgiveness. Who does confession benefit? In order to answer that question, turn to Psalm 32:1-2. What are the two benefits of forgiveness, according to those verses?

_____

_____

Now continue your reading of Psalm 32 through verses 3 and 4. What happened when David tried to cover up His sin rather than allow God to cover his sins through forgiveness?

_____

_____

_____

David's agony, as described in Psalm 32:3-4, was physical, mental, emotional and spiritual. List how David's lack of confession showed up in each of these areas of his being.

Physical: _____

_____

Mental: _____

_____

Emotional: _____

_____

Spiritual: _____

_____

How might God's hand being heavy on us because of unconfessed sin be one of the things that press in on us and keep us from pressing forward?

_____

_____

_____

Have you experienced unconfessed sin physically, mentally, emotionally or spiritually in your life—or all of the above? Explain your answer.

_____

_____

_____

Psalm 32:5 is good news indeed! What did David do, and what was the result of his action?

_____

_____

Carefully read Psalm 32:6-7. After David had experienced God's forgiveness, what did he express to God as part of his gratitude?

_____

_____

Some biblical scholars believe that the little word "selah" found in the margin of your Bible after verses 5 and 7 of Psalm 32 means "stop and think about it." Stop and think about how it feels to confess your sins and receive God's forgiveness. After you have pondered the awesome truths found in Psalm 32, write a prayer of thanksgiving to God for His mercy and compassion—and His forgiveness. Do your writing in your spiritual journal.

*O compassionate Father, I am indeed blessed because You are my God, the One who forgives all my sins. Amen.*

# HIDDEN BUT NOT COVERED UP

*O Lord, help me to never cover up my sins but instead to confess them to You so that I can be hidden with Christ in God. Amen.*

Yesterday our lesson explored the wonderful benefits of forgiveness. What did you learn that will encourage you to bring your sins to God rather than vainly try to cover them up?

_____

_____

_____

In Psalm 32:7, David calls God his "hiding place." What are the two benefits listed in Psalm 32:7 for taking refuge in God?

_____

_____

In order to understand the first benefit, being protected in times of trouble, look at the final section of Psalm 32:6. The rising waters are a symbol of final, absolute chaos that only God can overcome. Does "protect me from trouble" mean we will never have trials, hardships or troubles in this life? Why or why not?

_____

_____

_____

The second benefit of taking refuge in God is being surrounded with songs of deliverance. What are we delivered from, and why is this a reason to sing?

_____

_____

Our memory verse this week comes from chapter 3 of Colossians. Earlier in the week, we looked at the verses that come immediately before our memory verse. Now turn back to Colossians 3, this time concentrating on verses 2-3. What are we exhorted to do in these verses and why?

_____

_____

_____

How is being hidden with Christ in God like making God your hiding place?

How can being hidden with Christ be an important part of the First Place 4 Health program, and what is the self we must die to before that can happen?

When we are hidden with Christ in God, what happens to those things that press in on us and threaten our health and fitness goals?

Right after this week's memory verse, which is Colossians 3:14, Paul gives us another command. According to Colossians 3:15, what is to rule in our hearts?

How is having the peace of Christ in our hearts part of being hidden with Christ in God?

Peace is another of those virtues we usually apply to our relationships with others but not to our relationship with ourselves. What happens when the different parts of our being are at war with one another?

What happens when we devote our time and energy to our spiritual, mental and emotional health but neglect our physical health and fitness?

_____

_____

_____

How is the balance we find in the First Place 4 Health program an antidote to internal warfare?

_____

_____

_____

Can you really achieve wholeness and balance while you are mistreating your body, no matter how strong the other aspects of your First Place 4 Health program? Why or why not?

_____

_____

_____

*Thank You, loving Lord, for allowing me to hide myself with Christ in You. When the worries of this world press in on me, I will snuggle up closer to You. Amen.*

## Day 6 — REFLECTION AND APPLICATION

*My Lord and my God, help me to put off the things that keep me from putting on my new life in Christ Jesus, my Lord. Amen.*

During our Day Three study, we looked at Colossians 3:5-8 and the list of things Paul tells us we must put off so that we can put on Christ. Although we may not have been guilty of "sexual immorality, impurity, lust, evil desires and greed" mentioned in verse 5 (although in one form or another, we probably have done those things), all of us in First Place 4 Health have given in to our earthly nature when it comes to food. So today, instead of looking at Paul's list of vices, we are going to make our own.

In the left-hand column of the chart below, list your "binge foods"—those foods that you cannot moderate and must therefore eliminate from your food plan. Then, in the column on the right, list a healthy alternative you can eat in place of the foods that leave you heading for the cupboard and screaming, "More!"

| Binge Foods that Leave Me Crying for "More" | Healthy Foods that Satisfy |
|---|---|
|  |  |
|  |  |
|  |  |
|  |  |
|  |  |
|  |  |
|  |  |

How is eliminating your personal binge foods from your diet part of putting on the new self that is yours in Christ Jesus?

How does eliminating your personal binge foods allow you to move forward together with God in the First Place 4 Health program?

*Thank You, Father, for giving me the courage to be honest with myself about the foods that trigger out-of-control eating. Amen.*

## REFLECTION AND APPLICATION

*O Lord, I can only achieve unity with my brothers*
*and sisters when I am first unified within myself. Amen.*

"Every kingdom divided against itself will be ruined, and every city or household divided against itself will not stand," declared Jesus (Matthew 12:25). And that same principle of divided loyalties applies to our participation in First Place 4 Health. Listed below are the four aspects of a person. As you consider each side of you, describe how each part is at war or at peace with the other three when it comes to wholehearted commitment to First Place 4 Health. Usually when we are fragmented in our loyalties, either one part dominates or all parts fail. Identify which part of you dominates the others and which parts fail as a result. Or are the inner pieces of you in such discord that none of them can succeed? This exercise requires thought and honesty, so remember our lessons about confessing rather than covering up.

Physical: _____

_____

Mental: _____

_____

Emotional: _____

_____

Spiritual: _____

_____

What do you need to do to bind all four parts of you together in unity, which is the goal of balance that we strive for in First Place 4 Health?

_____

_____

_____

*O Lord God, help me to mend the broken pieces within me so that I can move forward together with You in love and unity. Amen.*

## *Group Prayer Requests*

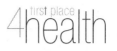

Today's Date: _____

| Name | Request |
|------|---------|
|      |         |
|      |         |
|      |         |
|      |         |
|      |         |
|      |         |
|      |         |
|      |         |
|      |         |
|      |         |

## Results

_____

_____

_____

_____

_____

_____

_____

# pursuit
# presses on

SCRIPTURE MEMORY VERSE

*But you, man of God, flee from all this, and pursue righteousness,*
*godliness, faith, love, endurance and gentleness.*

1 TIMOTHY 6:11

During last week's Bible study, we learned that it was necessary to put our Scripture memory verse into the larger Bible passage in which it appears before we can understand what the words of our memory verse are intended to teach. In order for us to put love above all the other virtues, we had to learn what "all" those virtues were!

Our memory verse last week is not an isolated example of the principle of Bible interpretation that looks to the surrounding text in order to correctly understand a specific verse. As a matter of fact, the "rule of five" is a good practice to remember: Read at least five verses *before* and five verses *after* a specific verse to properly understand what God is saying through that verse.

Sometimes proper understanding requires that we read the entire chapter in which the verse appears. At other times, especially when a chapter begins with the word "therefore," we need to go back to the previous chapter in order to understand what the word "therefore" is there for. To pull a verse out of context and then try to base our belief on a partial (or even incorrect) understanding of what is really being said in that verse is a grave error. Untold spiritual damage has been done because God's Word has not been considered in its entirety. Instead of drawing from the whole counsel of God, statements and judgments have been based on isolated verses pulled out of their proper context.

Our Week Six memory verse is another excellent example of the necessity of applying this basic principle of biblical interpretation. Write this week's memory verse, and then circle the words in this verse that tell us we need to read the verses that precede our memory verse in order to correctly understand this teaching.

_____

_____

_____

_____

## ALL THIS    Day 1

*Gracious God, You are the source of all wisdom and truth. Today I will listen to Your voice so that I will not be deceived by false teachings. Amen.*

"But you, man of God, flee from all this." With these words, the apostle Paul invites us to discover exactly what it is we are to flee from so that as a man or woman of God we can pursue the lifestyle that is pleasing to our Lord and Master. The first indication that we need to read the text that appears prior to this verse is the word "but"—a little conjunction that tells us our behavior is to be different from what has been described in previous verses. And as we saw in last week's memory verse, we must understand what "all this" is in order to flee from it! In order to fully understand what this verse is saying to us, we need to apply the "rule of five" mentioned in the introduction to this week's study. So let's go back five verses to Timothy 6:6 to see if we can learn what Paul is telling us we must avoid. Make special note of the word verse 6 begins with.

With the appearance of the conjunction "but," we know that we must go back a few verses further to understand this teaching. So let's begin our study by looking at 1 Timothy 6:3. Carefully read 1 Timothy 6:3-10, and in your own words, summarize what Paul says.

_____

_____

_____

What problem does Paul address in this passage?

_____

_____

_____

How might diet and exercise programs you participated in prior to coming to First Place 4 Health have been guilty of trying to make a profit but teaching a false truth that was not based on sound nutrition and exercise principles?

_____

_____

_____

Using the words of this week's memory verse as your example, what do you think the apostle Paul would say about such diet and exercise programs?

_____

_____

_____

What does this tell you about the importance of participating in a program with biblical integrity?

_____

_____

_____

*Thank You, sovereign Lord! In Your love and mercy, You brought me to First Place 4 Health. You saw my plight and allowed me to flee from the diet and exercise programs that were leading me down the wrong path. Amen.*

Day
2

## THE PRINCIPLE OF REPLACEMENT

*Gracious God, thank You for allowing me to replace my faulty beliefs and behavior with the tonic and truth of Your Word. Amen.*

During yesterday's lesson, we learned a foundational principle that will help us correctly interpret God's Word. Summarize what you learned about accurately understanding Scripture as you completed yesterday's Bible study lesson.

_____

_____

_____

Why is accurately understanding God's Word an important part of First Place 4 Health and moving forward toward your health and fitness goals?

_____

_____

_____

We must correctly understand what God is telling us if we hope to do things in a way that pleases Him and brings us blessing. Another important lesson we need to learn from Scripture is "the principle of replacement": We learn not only what things that erode our spiritual growth and development need to be eliminated from our lives, but we also learn what life-sustaining choices should replace those bad habits. Last week's Bible study is a good example of this principle. What were we told to take off so that we could put on the new person we are becoming in Christ Jesus?

_____

_____

_____

We also see the principle of replacement played out in the passage from 1 Timothy that contains this week's memory verse. Carefully reread 1 Timothy 6:3-10, and list the things the apostle Paul admonishes us to flee from. There are many, so list as many as you can find.

_____

_____

_____

According to 1 Timothy 6:3-10, what life-giving behaviors are we to put in place of the things we are to flee from?

_____

_____

_____

Finally, In 1 Timothy 6:11 (this week's memory verse), Paul lists the desirable virtues that are to replace the vices that describe people with corrupt minds. What virtues are we told to pursue?

_____

_____

_____

Review your list of the things our memory verse tells us to flee from, and identify one behavior or belief that you need to replace with a life-giving behavior or belief. Discuss why you selected this particular item as something you need to flee from, and describe how this negative trait impacts your First Place 4 Health program.

_____

_____

_____

_____

Which of the virtues Paul encourages us to pursue can you use to replace that negative behavior or belief, and why?

_____

_____

_____

_____

What can you do _today_ to flee from the thing that keeps you from moving forward so that you can pursue the lifestyle God is calling you to in First Place 4 Health?

_____

_____

_____

_____

_O gracious and loving God, You not only show me what is damaging, but You also show me life-sustaining ways that allow me to press forward toward the prize You have for me in First Place 4 Health. Amen._

## O MAN OF GOD

*O Lord God, what a profound privilege it is to be*
*called a servant of the true and living God. Amen.*

During this week's Bible study lessons, we have learned about some foundational principles that prepare us to press on toward the prize. One of these principles is the "rule of five." What is "the rule of five," and why is it important to our First Place 4 Health journey?

We have already read the verses preceding this week's memory verse. What did you learn from reading 1 Timothy 6:3-10 that helped you better understand what we are being taught in our memory verse?

But the "rule of five" doesn't stop with just reading the verses that come before the verse we are striving to better understand. We must also read the five verses after the verse. Read 1 Timothy 6:12-16. What information in these verses gives you more insight into the meaning of this week's memory verse?

Write out this week's memory verse, and underline the words Paul uses to describe Timothy in this passage.

What information do you find in 1 Timothy 6:12-16 that helps you better understand what it means to be a man or woman of God?

What is the "good confession" Timothy had made in the presence of many witnesses (verse 12)? (Romans 10:9-13 will help you with this answer.)

_____

_____

Why do you think that it was important that Timothy had made his profession of faith in the presence of many witnesses rather than just being a "secret service" Christian?

_____

_____

Recall the time you made your profession of faith in the presence of many witnesses. How have you grown in grace and knowledge since the moment you invited Jesus Christ to be the Lord and Savior of your life?

_____

_____

Is there really such a thing as a "secret service" Christian? Why or why not?

_____

_____

_____

(_Note:_ If you have not made a public profession of faith and would like to do so, please talk to your First Place 4 Health leader, a pastor or spiritual director, or a mature Christian friend. They can help you make a profession that supports your faith journey.)

If the apostle Paul were writing you a letter, could he truthfully refer to you as a man or woman of God? Why or why not? Please give concrete evidence to support your answer.

_____

_____

_____

Would your friends and coworkers agree that you are indeed a man or woman of God? Or would they be surprised to hear you addressed that way? Why?

_____

_____

_____

_____

How has the First Place 4 Health program been part of your good confession and your growth in grace and knowledge?

_____

_____

_____

*O gracious and loving Master, sometimes it is difficult to live my confession of faith in front of others who do not believe in You. Forgive me for those times I think I can go underground and serve You in secret. Amen.*

## IN GOD'S OWN TIME — Day 4

*Dear Lord, help me to "fight the good fight" and press on when I am feeling discouraged. Thank You that You are the One who gives life to all things. Amen.*

Yesterday we began to study the verses that come right after this week's memory verse. What did you learn from that study?

_____

_____

_____

Today we are going to continue the study we began yesterday. Reread 1 Timothy 6:12-16. Why are we reading these particular verses?

_____

_____

_____

In 1 Timothy 6:12, Paul tells Timothy to _____ the good _____ .
How does this admonition confirm what Paul is telling Timothy to do in our
memory verse?

_____

_____

_____

Although this letter was written to Timothy, it is applicable to all who strive to
live a life worthy of the title "Man (or Woman) of God." What do the words "fight
the good fight" mean to you as they apply to your First Place 4 Health program?

_____

_____

_____

How is fighting the good fight like pressing on toward the prize?

_____

_____

In what appears to be a contradiction in terms, Paul tells us to flee so that we
can fight. How is fleeing from the things that keep us pressed down part of
fighting "the good fight of faith" (1 Timothy 6:12)?

_____

_____

_____

Paul tells us to press on in the sight of God—the One who gives life to everything.
If you were always mindful that God gave life to your body and that you are always in God's sight, how would the way you care for your body be impacted?

_____

_____

_____

In 1 Timothy 6:14, we are told how long we are to fight the good fight of faith.
How long are we to continue to press on?

_____

_____

Who knows exactly the day and hour when Jesus Christ will appear, and when will this glorious event come to pass? (First Timothy 6:15 has both answers.)

What does this tell you about the nature of the journey to health and wholeness that we are making in the First Place 4 Health program?

In 1 Timothy 6:14, Paul tells us to keep the commandment "without spot or blemish." But often we fail to keep the commandment perfectly. Who is the One without spot or blemish who perfectly kept the Law for us so that we could be made perfect in His righteousness? (Read 1 Peter 1:18-19, if you need help with the answer.)

The same "rule of five" that tells us to read five verses before and five verses after the passage we are striving to better understand also has another "five" component: Meditate on the passage for five minutes. Spend the rest of your quiet time meditating on the truths you have learned in today's study.

> *O Lord God, thank You for sending Jesus, the Lamb without spot or defect, to perfectly keep the Law so that I can be perfect in His righteousness. Amen.*

## KING OF KINGS AND LORD OF LORDS

**Day 5**

*O Lord, may the words of my mouth and the meditations of my heart be pleasing in your sight, my Rock and my Redeemer. Amen* (Psalm 19:14).

At the end of yesterday's lesson, we learned that in addition to reading five verses before the passage we are studying and then reading five verses after the passage we are studying, the rule of five has a third component. What is that third component?

_____

_____

How is this like the little word "selah" that we saw at the end of Psalm 32:5 and 7?

_____

_____

Selah invites us to "take five" and stop and think about what we have just read! And that is exactly what the apostle Paul does at the end of the 1 Timothy 6 passage we have been studying this week. For our benefit, Paul wrote his meditation down. Turn to 1 Timothy 6:15-16. Paul began this passage by telling us that God will bring about the second coming of Jesus in _____ own _____. The words that follow this clearly indicate that Paul's mind and heart are swept up in a wonderful benediction-type prayer. How do we know these words are a meditation? (The last word of verse 16 holds the answer.)

_____

_____

In 1 Timothy 6:15, Paul uses several words to describe the God he is meditating on. What are those words?

_____

_____

Following the description of God, Paul gives us some additional information about this God who is the blessed and only Ruler, the King of kings and Lord of lords. What three bits of information about God does Paul give us in 1 Timothy 6:16?

_____

_____

_____

In light of who God is, what does Paul tell us He is deserving of? (The end of 1 Timothy 6:16 has the answer.)

_____

_____

And for how long is our God to receive honor and might?

_____

_____

What can you learn about how we are to "take five" in meditation from reading Paul's wonderful words?

_____

_____

How is meditating on who God is and what He has done for us part of the First Place 4 Health program?

_____

_____

How is meditating on who God is and what He has done for us part of pressing on toward the prize and fleeing from the things that keep us enslaved to destructive beliefs and behaviors?

_____

_____

Pick one of Paul's statements about God from today's study and write a meditation on that aspect of God's character and nature. Use your spiritual journal for this exercise.

_O Lord God, when I consider who You are, I stand in awe that You love and care for me. Amen._

## REFLECTION AND APPLICATION

*Faithful Father, thank You for teaching me how to read and meditate on Your Word through this Bible study. Amen.*

One of the Scripture-interpretation principles we have learned during this week's Bible study is called the "rule of five" (so appropriate for our fifth week study!). What three components of the "rule of five" have we learned about so far?

_____

_____

_____

As the name implies, there are actually five components to the "rule of five," leaving two parts of this important principle we have not yet learned about. The fourth aspect of the "rule of five" is to read out loud five times a day the verse being studied. How would this aspect of the "rule of five" help you memorize Scripture?

_____

_____

_____

Write this week's memory verse on a small index card or use the Scripture memory cards provided in the back of this study. Having the verse on a portable medium will allow you to carry it with you so that you can say the verse out loud at various times during the day.

How can the four components of the "rule of five" that we have learned thus far be incorporated into your First Place 4 Health practice?

_____

_____

_____

How is the "rule of five" part of pressing on toward the prize and fighting the good fight?

_____

_____

_____

*O Lord God Almighty, You ask that I hide Your Word in my heart so that I won't sin against You. Help me to read and meditate on Your Word so that I can both memorize and apply the lessons You have for me to my life. Amen (Psalm 119:11).*

## REFLECTION AND APPLICATION

**Day 7**

*Lord God Almighty, all true learning results in application. Help me, gracious God, to apply what I have learned this week to my First Place 4 Health efforts. Amen.*

Today we will learn about the fifth component of the "rule of five." As we begin this day of reflection and application, please list the four components of the "rule of five" we have already learned. Leave the fifth line blank for now.

1. _____

2. _____

3. _____

4. _____

5. _____

The fifth part of the "rule of five" is the application part of the learning process. It asks us to identify five ways we can apply the verse we are studying to our life in a very practical way. Add "Apply the verse five ways" to the list above. Next, write this week's memory verse. You should be able to write it from memory by now!

_____

_____

_____

Think about ways you can apply the words of this verse to your daily First Place 4 Health lifestyle. The applications can be implied in the verse itself, but think of ways that are practical—and doable! As you go about your day, begin applying your ideas to your beliefs and behavior.

*My Lord and my God, all too often I talk about what I am going to do. I make lists and more lists, but somehow they don't become part of my daily beliefs and behaviors. Help me, Lord, to actually apply the words I have written today to my First Place 4 Health program. Amen.*

## *Group Prayer Requests*

Today's Date: _____

| Name | Request |
|------|---------|
|      |         |
|      |         |
|      |         |
|      |         |
|      |         |
|      |         |
|      |         |
|      |         |
|      |         |

## Results

_____

_____

_____

_____

_____

_____

*Week Seven*

# all who run can win

SCRIPTURE MEMORY VERSE
*Do you not know that in a race all the runners run, but only one gets the prize?*
*Run in such a way as to get the prize.*
1 CORINTHIANS 9:24

Wow! We have crossed the halfway mark in our Bible study, and we have covered a lot of ground! Using the little word "selah" we learned about in our Week Five study and the "take five" principle we learned about last week, take some time to recap the major points you have learned in each week's study. You will probably want to review each week's lessons in order to refresh your memory.

Week Two:

_____

_____

_____

Week Three:

_____

_____

_____

Week Four:

_____

_____

_____

Week Five:

_____

_____

_____

Week Six:

_____

_____

_____

How have you been able to apply these lessons in concrete ways to your First Place 4 Health program?

_____

_____

_____

_____

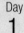

Day
1

## COMPETITION

*Gracious God, thank You for giving us examples we can easily understand so that we can take Your Word to heart and apply it in meaningful ways to our First Place 4 Health journey. Amen.*

The ancient Greeks held four national festivals (or games) in which athletes competed for a prize. The most popular of these national events, the Olympic Games, has been revived in modern times. The Isthmian Games were the next in popularity among the Greek national festivals, and these competitions were held on the Isthmus of Corinth every two years. Because the Corinthians were well acquainted with these Isthmian Games, the apostle Paul used the analogy of a runner competing for the prize when writing to the saints at Corinth about how to live a life pleasing to God. What spiritual truth is Paul teaching us by using the example of a runner in this week's memory verse?

_____

_____

_____

When Jesus was here on Earth, He taught in parables, earthly stories that the common people of His day could easily understand. How is Paul's use of competing for the prize like Jesus' teaching in parables?

What does this tell you about God's desire to communicate with us in a way we can readily understand?

How is pressing on part of running in a way that will win the prize that awaits us as we are faithful to the First Place 4 Health program?

In this week's memory verse, Paul tells us that in a race, _____ the _____ run, but only _____ gets the _____. But when it comes to the prize that awaits us in First Place 4 Health, does only one person reach his or her goal while the rest must settle for second, third or even last place? Explain your answer.

Who is it that we compete against in First Place 4 Health: the other members of our group, knowing we can only win if they lose; or our own personal best, striving to improve our performance while encouraging our companions to do their personal best? How can you use the analogy of a runner competing in the games as you strive to achieve your own personal best in First Place 4 Health?

*Gracious and loving God, I am so thankful that I do not need to compete against my brothers and sisters in Christ. Your love and grace are not extended to only those who can run the fastest, but rather to all who call on Your name and look to You for salvation. Amen.*

## Day 2 — FREEDOM TO BE FAITHFUL

*Dear Lord, thank You for the strength You have given to me in the First Place 4 Health program. Let me share the blessing of the gospel with others. Amen.*

Last week we learned many points to remember about Scripture interpretation that will help us run in such a way as to win the prize. Those points concerned the "rule of five." What is the first component of the "rule of five"?

Today, as we strive to better understand what is being said in this week's memory verse, let's turn to 1 Corinthians 9 and read verses 19-23, the five verses before our memory verse. Read those verses carefully, and then summarize what they teach us.

Earlier in 1 Corinthians 9, the apostle Paul declared that he was "compelled to preach . . . the gospel" (1 Corinthians 9:16). How is Paul putting his words into practice in 1 Corinthians 9:19-23?

How does reading 1 Corinthians 9:19-23 help you understand why Paul chose to use the analogy of a runner in his teaching?

How are you called to preach the good news of Jesus Christ through participation in the First Place 4 Health program, especially as it applies to reaching out to those who suffer from the consequences of out-of-control eating?

_____

_____

_____

_____

Just as Paul gave substance to his declaration that he was compelled to preach the gospel, what are you doing to put into practice your words about reaching out to others?

_____

_____

_____

_____

In 1 Corinthians 9:23, Paul says he does all this "for the _____ of the _____ , that _____ may _____ in its blessing." How are you sharing in the blessing of the gospel when you reach out to others in need of First Place 4 Health?

_____

_____

_____

_____

Paul says he became weak in order to win the weak (see 1 Corinthians 9:22). How is admitting your weakness—and the strength you have found through Christ in First Place 4 Health—part of becoming weak in order to win the weak?

_____

_____

_____

_____

Think of one person who is still being held in bondage to out-of-control eating, and look for an opportunity to share the good news of First Place 4 Health with that individual. You will be telling your First Place 4 Health group how you fulfilled this assignment at your next meeting, so take action rather than settle for good intentions. Briefly describe your experience here so that you'll be able to recall the details at the meeting.

_____

_____

_____

> *O Lord, although I may not be called to preach the gospel like Paul, I am called to share the good news I have found in You. Help me to be a faithful witness. Amen.*

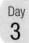

## Day 3 — TRAINING, TRAINING, TRAINING

*Lord, help me to stay focused as I train to gain endurance physically, mentally, emotionally and spiritually. Amen.*

Having completed the first component of the "rule of five," our next assignment is to read the _____ verses _____ our memory verse. However, as there are only 27 verses in 1 Corinthians 9, we will conclude our reading at the chapter's end. But before turning to 1 Corinthians 9:25-27, write out this week's memory verse so that it will be fresh in your mind during today's study.

_____

_____

_____

What does Paul tell us that all those who compete in the games do before the competition? (The answer is in 1 Corinthians 9:25.)

_____

_____

_____

What type of training are you currently doing that will give you the strength and endurance necessary to complete the course set before you? First Place 4 Health emphasizes training in all four aspects of our being, so list the training you are doing in each area. Then, for each type of training you list, describe how each type of training is part of the preparation you will need if you are going to press on toward the prize.

Physically: _____

_____

Mentally: _____

_____

Emotionally: _____

_____

Spiritually: _____

_____

Look at the chart below that lists the aspects of the four-sided person. In which two areas do you have the most strength, and why do you think that is so? Which two areas are the weakest, and why do you think that is so?

_____

_____

_____

| PHYSICAL | MENTAL |
|----------|--------|
| EMOTIONAL | SPIRITUAL |

Using Paul's analogy, picture an athlete trying to compete in a race when half of his or her body is considerably stronger than the other half. What would be the result?

_____

_____

Likewise, what happens to your ability to press on toward the prize when your strength is not equally balanced?

_____

_____

_____

What do you need to do to bring balance to your First Place 4 Health efforts so that you will not grow weary and lose heart during the journey that lies ahead of you?

_____

_____

_____

_____

*Father God, I know I am only as strong as my weakest part. Help me to achieve the balance and wholeness that honors You. Amen.*

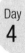

Day
4

## MOTIVATED TO WIN

*Gracious Lord, how often I devote my time and energy to things that do not have lasting value. Help me to store up treasures in heaven, not expend my resources on things that have no eternal value. Amen* (Luke 12:33).

Yesterday we began to look at the verses that immediately follow our memory verse for Week Seven. Reread 1 Corinthians 9:24-27 in your Bible (our memory verse and the remainder of the verses in 1 Corinthians 9). Did the Holy Spirit bring any words to your attention that you missed in yesterday's reading?

_____

_____

_____

In yesterday's study of 1 Corinthians 9:25, we learned that all athletes go into strict training before they enter a competition. What did you learn about your First Place 4 Health training endeavors from that study?

_____

_____

_____

Those who are training to run in an actual physical race train for one specific reason. What does Paul tell us is the motivation of those who run in the Isthmian Games? (First Corinthians 9:25 has the answer.)

_____

_____

_____

How is the motivation different for those of us who are in training to run the spiritual race that leads us heavenward in Christ Jesus?

_____

_____

_____

What is the difference between the two prizes? (You might want to look at Jesus' words in Matthew 6:19-21 as you contemplate your answer.)

_____

_____

_____

What determines our motivation, the prize we are willing to work for?

_____

_____

_____

How is the First Place 4 Health program part of storing up treasures in heaven rather than competing for an earthly crown?

_____

_____

_____

What will happen if our motivation is to achieve physical results in First Place 4 Health but the spiritual dimension is missing?

_____

_____

_____

What will happen if we concentrate on the spiritual component of First Place 4 Health but neglect the physical component? (Yesterday's lesson on balance will help you answer this question.)

According to 1 Corinthians 9:26, what is Paul not doing?

If we are not focused on the prize, we will run aimlessly. How does your weekly First Place 4 Health group meeting help you to stay focused on what is important?

How is using lots of boastful words that are not followed by consistent action like beating the air?

Does your First Place 4 Health training regime more closely resemble that of a serious athlete or that of one running aimlessly, and why?

*O Lord God, how thankful I am that I can store up treasures in heaven rather than competing with those who are focused on earthly gain. Amen.*

## SELF-DISCIPLINE Day **5**

*O Lord, Your Word is truth; it is only my faulty perceptions that cause confusion.*
*Help me understand what You would have me learn through today's lesson. Amen.*

It is important to read particular passages of Scripture in the light of the full counsel of God's Word. Paul uses such athletic imagery as found in 1 Corinthians 9:27 throughout his writing, and Philippians 3:12, a verse that is part of the same passage as our Week Two memory verse, is another example. Turn to that verse now and look at the use of the words "take hold." What is Paul striving to take hold of, and who has taken hold of Paul?

_____

_____

_____

We see that same writing technique used in 1 Corinthians 9:26-27. How does Paul use the word "beat" in these two verses?

_____

_____

But when Paul says he "beats" his body, he is not talking about self-abuse! He is using the word "beat" to speak of the loving self-discipline that he must apply if he is going to run the same race he is encouraging others to run. How do we know this is so? Turn to 1 Corinthians 9:27. What does this verse tell us?

_____

_____

_____

Now turn to 1 Corinthians 3:16-17. What do these verses teach us?

_____

_____

_____

How does looking at other passages of Scripture help clarify what Paul is really saying in 1 Corinthians 9:27?

What can you learn from this exercise that will help you correctly understand other difficult passages in Scripture?

How is loving self-discipline part of the First Place 4 Health program?

Is anything in First Place 4 Health abusive to your body, or does First Place 4 Health reinforce the spiritual principle of caring for God's temple, your physical self? Explain your answer.

In 1 Corinthians 9:27, Paul says he has made his body his slave—his servant. How can we use loving self-discipline so that our body serves us well and allows us to run the race set before us in First Place 4 Health?

What have you learned during today's lesson that will help you flee from the faulty beliefs and behaviors that keep you from running in such a way as to get the prize?

_____

_____

_____

*Gracious and loving Lord, thank You for giving me the ability to be a worker approved by You, for me to be one who knows how to correctly handle the truth found in Your Word. Amen.*

## REFLECTION AND APPLICATION

Day 6

*Mighty and merciful God, today I thank You for leading me in right paths and for putting my feet on firm ground. Jesus died for me; it is my desire to live for You. Amen.*

A story is told about a young high school athlete who was preparing to represent his school in the high-jump event at a state-level championship meet. His school was favored in many of the track and field events, and this young man had set his heart on being part of the team of athletes that would bring honor to their school on that day. For months the young man practiced, and for months the young man's coach consistently raised the bar to a higher level as the jumper's proficiency increased. As the day of the competition approached, the coach put the bar up to the state record-breaking height for that event.

"Aw, come on, Coach, I'll never be able to jump that high!" sighed the young man.

"Just throw your heart over the bar first, and before you know it, the rest of you will follow," replied the coach.

And the coach was right; the young man went on to set a new state record because he had thrown his heart over the bar, confident that his body would follow where his heart had gone first.

And so it is with us in our First Place 4 Health endeavors. Little by little, our Master Coach and Personal Trainer, Jesus, continues to raise the bar and encourage us to grow in our faith. And like the young athlete, we must send our heart ahead of us if we hope to run the race in a way that will lead us to our desired destination.

How has God raised the bar for you since you first began this session of First Place 4 Health?

How has the training you have been doing in all four aspects of your being helped you to successfully navigate the obstacles you have faced during this session of First Place 4 Health?

Have you completely "thrown your heart over the bar" so that your body can follow, or are you still looking at other weight-loss alternatives that you feel might help you attain your goal faster than the sure, steady, lifelong progress that is part of the First Place 4 Health journey?

*Lord God, I know that in those areas that I have not thrown my heart over the bar, I resemble the racer who runs aimlessly. You desire wholehearted devotion, not half measures that do not result in First Place 4 Health progress. Amen.*

## Day 7 — REFLECTION AND APPLICATION

*Faithful Father, You ask that I love You with all my heart, mind, body and spirit. Today I will honor You by exercising the wonderfully made body You created and called good. Amen.*

This week's study used a runner to teach us about the importance of training ourselves to run as one who will get the prize. So today we are going to go out and do some multi-purpose First Place 4 Health training. Wear your athletic shoes and bring along the Scripture memory card containing this week's memory verse.

As you begin to walk, start repeating this week's Scripture memory verse in cadence with your steps. Each time you repeat the memory verse, emphasize a different word in the verse, using both your voice and your footsteps to accentuate the word. Begin by emphasizing the first word in the memory verse. The next time you say the verse emphasize the second word, the next time the third word, and so on until you have gone through the verse 28 times, because there are 28 words that need to be accentuated during this training exercise.

Make a mental note of the different feels the verse has as each different word in the verse is stressed both physically and verbally. When you return home, write down in your prayer journal any new insights the Holy Spirit brought to your awareness as you emphasized each word in the verse in cadence with your steps. For your next First Place 4 Health group meeting, be prepared to give a report on what you experienced during this exercise.

*O Lord, it is good to walk in sync with Your Word. Thank You for sending the Holy Spirit to guide my steps and enlighten my mind as I meditate on the lessons You have for me. Amen.*

## Group Prayer Requests

4 first place
health

Today's Date: _____

| Name | Request |
|------|---------|
|      |         |
|      |         |
|      |         |
|      |         |
|      |         |
|      |         |
|      |         |
|      |         |
|      |         |
|      |         |

## Results

_____

_____

_____

_____

_____

_____

# true glory

SCRIPTURE MEMORY VERSE
*When the Chief Shepherd appears,*
*you will receive the crown of glory that will never fade away.*
1 PETER 5:4

Although runners competing in the Isthmian Games underwent rigorous physical training to increase their speed and endurance in preparation for the big event, the runners were not just judged on speed; they were also judged on form. Yes, winning was important, but how one ran—sportsmanship—was also part of the competition. Did runners stay in their proper lane? Did they cut off fellow runners? Did they compete by the established rules for that event? All this was part of walking away with the prize.

Even now, our modern Olympic Games still retain vestiges of the dual emphases stressed in the original Greek games; running rightly is as important as running swiftly, and using proper form is an important part of winning the coveted gold medal. Yet for all their training, for all their self-discipline, for all their playing the game according to the rules, the athletes of the early Greek games were competing to win a wreath made of laurel leaves and a first-place title that would last only until the next event—when a younger, swifter runner would likely upstage the present champion.

How is running the Christian race different from physical competition, where youth and speed are usually the determining factors in the victory?

_____

_____

_____

_____

Yes, in the physical realm our bodies grow slower as they mature. Time takes away the professional athlete's competitive edge. Our aging bodies are more prone to injury, and our recovery time is longer with each passing year. Soon, younger athletes and more-advanced training methods move the next generation into the winner's circle; the older athletes retire from formal competition. However, in the spiritual realm, as we mature, we grow in grace and knowledge. As we saw in our Week Three study of Abraham and Sarah, even in our old age we can produce abundant fruit for our Master. Spiritual maturity is both a goal and a virtue in God's kingdom. No matter what our chronological age, we begin our journey of faith as infants, advance to spiritual adolescence and finally become mature mothers and fathers of the faith.

How is growing in grace and knowledge part of the First Place 4 Health program, and what benefit does spiritual maturity bring to our efforts?

_____

_____

_____

**Day 1**

## INSTRUCTIONS TO ELDERS

*O Lord God, You are the Chief Shepherd. Help me to hear Your voice and follow where You lead. Amen.*

The young emerging Church was beset by many problems. Converts from pagan religions were trying to blend their old beliefs with their new life in Christ. False teachers had infiltrated the flock of Jesus Christ, and their heresy was a constant threat to God's chosen people. Recall from your Week Six study the advice the apostle Paul gave young Timothy about fleeing from false teachers who were more interested in financial gain than preaching the truth of God's Word. Reread 1 Timothy 6:10. What does Paul say about people eager for money in this verse?

_____

_____

_____

The new churches founded by the apostle Paul weren't the only ones dealing with those who were greedy for money. The apostle Peter also wrote about this "greedy for money" problem in the passage this week's memory verse is taken from. Turn to 1 Peter 5:1-4 in your Bible, and read what Peter has to say.

Why is reading the text that comes before our Scripture memory verse important to our proper understanding of the truth contained in the verse we are committing to memory?

In 1 Peter 5:1, we learn exactly who Peter is addressing in this passage. To whom is this portion of Peter's epistle addressed?

How does Peter describe himself in 1 Peter 5:1?

What is the appeal Peter makes to these elders, and why did Peter specifically write to them?

In 1 Peter 5:2-3, the apostle gives the elders, who are the ones chosen to shepherd God's flock, some specific instructions. Paraphrase Peter's words.

How can Peter's words to the elders in the Early Church be incorporated into your First Place 4 Health program?

If your First Place 4 Health group leader is not being an example to the little flock under his or her care, is that person qualified to be the leader of your group, regardless of his or her other qualifications for leadership? Explain your answer.

_____

_____

_____

*Gracious and loving Lord, thank You for giving me elders, those people who are mature in their faith and able to set an example for me. Amen.*

## Day 2 — TRUE GLORY

*O Lord God, there is no glory in this earth except the glory I find in my relationship with You. Amen.*

Yesterday we began to study 1 Peter 5:1-4, which is the passage in which we find this week's memory verse. Before we begin today's lesson, summarize what you learned yesterday from the apostle Peter's words.

_____

_____

_____

Our memory verse for this week talks about the reason elders are to be diligent in caring for the flock God has entrusted to their care. Why are they to be eager to serve and be living examples to their flock?

_____

_____

_____

Think back to the laurel-leaf wreath the Olympic Game runners received and to the fading glory of a winner's title that will all too soon go to another athlete. What does 1 Peter 5:4 tell us those who have faithfully served their Lord and Master will receive?

_____

_____

_____

Jesus is the Chief Shepherd (see John 10:11). How is Jesus' willingness to lay down His life for His flock different from those leaders in the Early Church who served for financial gain and lorded their position of authority over the people entrusted to their care (described in 1 Peter 5:2-3)?

_____

_____

_____

Recall from our Week Six study exactly when the Chief Shepherd will appear with the crown of glory that will not fade away. (First Timothy 6:14-15 has the answer, if you would like to refresh your memory.)

_____

_____

_____

Long before Peter and Paul wrote their epistles to the Early Church, the prophet Jeremiah talked about the source of our true glory: the crown that will never fade away. Turn to Jeremiah 9:23-24. What are the three things our Lord, through Jeremiah, tells us are not to be sources of boasting and pride?

1. _____

2. _____

3. _____

Based on Jeremiah 9:23 and the things you have learned in our Bible study, how can these three things be a detriment to our First Place 4 Health journey?

Boasting about our own wisdom:

_____

_____

Boasting about our own strength:

_____

_____

_____

Boasting about our financial position:

_____

_____

_____

How do these three things correspond to the things Paul told young Timothy to flee from in 1 Timothy 6:3-10? (Refer to our Week Six study, if you need help with the answer.)

_____

_____

_____

Jeremiah 9:24 tells us there is only one thing we have to boast about. What is it?

_____

_____

_____

How is First Place 4 Health part of understanding and knowing God?

_____

_____

_____

What does God tell us about Himself in Jeremiah 9:24?

_____

_____

_____

How are kindness, justice and righteousness part of the exercise that allows you to run the race with proper form that produces spiritual maturity?

_____

_____

_____

_O sovereign Lord, You are the only One deserving of glory, honor and praise. Thank You for calling me into an intimate relationship with You so that I do not need to place undue value on the fleeting things of this world. Amen._

## ADVICE FOR THE YOUNG

*Merciful Father, You call me to live a life pleasing to You. Help me to study Your Word diligently and apply it faithfully to the daily events of my life. Amen.*

Our Week Six memory verse came from a letter the apostle Paul wrote to young Timothy, his disciple in the faith. What was the advice Paul gave Timothy in that verse? (Write the verse from memory; if you've forgotten the verse, turn to the verse in your Bible so that you can copy it.)

Paul also wrote a second letter to Timothy. In that epistle, Paul talked to Timothy about the importance of a type of training that is not physical in nature. Read 2 Timothy 2:15. What does Paul encourage young Timothy to do?

How is learning how to correctly handle the Word of God part of fleeing from things that have the potential to keep you from pressing on toward the prize?

One of the ways we have learned to correctly handle God's Word through our Bible study is to read verses before and after the specific verse we are studying so that we can understand what is really being taught. What is the danger of pulling verses out of the passage in which they were written and trying to build our faith on those one or two sentences pulled out of context?

In keeping with the practice of sound Bible interpretation, let's read the verses that Peter wrote right after he addressed the elders in the Church with specific instructions for the way they were to shepherd the flock God had entrusted to their care. Turn to 1 Peter 5:5-9 in your Bible. To whom is this portion of Peter's letter addressed?

_____

_____

Do you think those are young men (and women) chronologically or spiritually? Consider the example of young Timothy, who was an elder in the Church, as you answer this question.

_____

_____

_____

Just as the elders are to submit to the Lordship of the Chief Shepherd, who are the younger Christians in the flock to submit to?

_____

_____

What have the leaders done to be deserving of that respect? (Refer to 1 Peter 5:3 for the answer, and also consider whom the leaders are accountable to as you answer this question.)

_____

_____

What else does Paul tell the younger Christians to do in 1 Peter 5:5, and why does Peter tell them to do so?

_____

_____

_____

During our Week Five Bible study, we learned about some multi-purpose, one-size-fits-all clothing Christians are to put on. How do Peter's words in 1 Peter 5:5 affirm that earlier teaching?

As we look at 1 Peter 5:6-7, we see Peter talking about humbling ourselves under God's hand and casting our cares on Him because He cares for us. How is casting your cares on God an act of humility?

What are we told to do in 1 Peter 5:8-9? Summarize in your own words what Peter teaches in these verses.

How is resisting the devil so that you can stand firm in your faith like fleeing from the things that keep you from leading a godly life?

We have learned many important spiritual principles in today's study. What one specific thing have you learned that will help you move forward in your First Place 4 Health efforts?

*Loving Father, today I will humble myself under Your mighty hand, confident that You care for me and will never do anything to harm me when I submit myself to Your authority. Amen.*

Day
4

# THE MASTER'S JOY

*O Lord God, how glorious will be the day when You return to reward Your faithful, fruitful servants and allow them to enter into Your joy. Amen.*

Paul and Peter used analogies about athletes, particularly the crowns and prizes athletes could win, to teach their disciples about living the Christian life. However, Jesus, the Chief Shepherd and overseer of the flock, did not talk about prizes or crowns. Jesus talked about bearing crosses and serving the Master. Turn to Matthew 25:14-30 in your Bible to read a parable Jesus told His disciples to explain what will happen when He comes again in glory to reward the faithful.

Although there are many lessons we can learn from this wonderful parable, to-day we will focus our attention on the reward we will receive when our Master returns. Two of the servants in this parable had been faithful and fruitful. What do verses 21 and 23 teach us about the reward we will get when the Master comes back for an accounting of the things entrusted to our care?

Does the Master give the faithful, fruitful servants a crown or a prize, like an athlete might receive after successfully completing a race? If not, what does He give them instead?

The Master praises them for their faithfulness and then tells them what being faithful in a few things will result in. According to Matthew 25:21, what will be given to those who have been faithful with a few things?

If Jesus were to return tonight and ask for an accounting of how you have managed the body He has entrusted to your care, would you be commended for being faithful in the little everyday things that comprise the First Place 4 Health program? Why or why not?

In addition to being put in charge of many things, the faithful, fruitful servants will be invited to do what when the Master appears (see Matthew 25:21)?

Read Hebrews 12:1-2. In verse 2, we are exhorted to look to Jesus, "the author and perfecter of our faith," as we run the race before us. Why did Jesus endure the cross, scorning its shame, according to Hebrews 12:2?

How is the anticipation of entering into the Master's happiness the same as enduring for the joy set before us?

What happened after Jesus endured the cross in anticipation of the joy that was before Him? (Hebrews 12:2 has the answer.)

How is persevering in anticipation of entering the Master's happiness, where there will be eternal joy, different from running to win a prize? Please give this question very careful thought!

Which reward is more appealing to you: a crown-type prize, or entering into your Master's happiness and being given more responsibility? Explain why you chose your answer.

_O Lord, so often we think in terms of a reward rather than following Your example and being faithful because it brings You joy. Forgive us for being so self-focused that we forget about You. Amen._

## Day 5

## BY GRACE ALONE

_O Lord God, I know there is nothing I can do to be deserving of Your love and grace. They are a free gift to me, no matter how well I run or how fiercely I compete in the game. Amen._

Although the image of receiving prizes and crowns is useful when it comes to teaching us how to live the Christian life with regard to training and focus, that same analogy can lead us into faulty thinking as it applies to our ability to earn salvation. Once again, it is essential that we weigh all the references to running and competing in light of the whole counsel of God! While Olympic-type runners run the course in their own strength and power, we do not. We can only run as God Himself empowers us to run. And although an Olympian can win a prize by sheer will and determination, we are powerless to save ourselves, let alone win a prize, when it comes to running the Christian race. Perhaps that is why the apostle Peter concluded chapter 5 of his first letter with a wonderful benediction that reminds us we are saved by grace and grace alone. Turn to 1 Peter 5:10-11 in your Bible, and read Peter's powerful words.

How does 1 Peter 5:10 describe God, and what does it say God has done for us?

Now let's read the words of the apostle Paul to learn more about the marvelous grace of God! Turn to Ephesians 2:4-10, and then summarize the verses in your own words.

_____

_____

_____

Is there any way we can work for, or earn, our own salvation, no matter how well we run the race? (Reread Ephesians 2:8-9 for the answer.)

_____

_____

_____

If we can't work for (or earn) our salvation, how is salvation granted, according to Ephesians 2:8?

_____

_____

_____

Who is it that raises us up and seats us in the heavenly realms with Christ Jesus? (Look to Ephesians 2:6 for the answer.)

_____

_____

_____

According to Ephesians 2:7, why did God do this?

_____

_____

_____

Ephesians 2:4 tells us God is rich in mercy. How was that mercy manifest, according to Ephesians 2:5?

_____

_____

_____

Because we do not work for our salvation, we have no reason to boast. Instead, we are called to respond to God's grace by doing good works (see Ephesians 2:10). We don't work *for* our salvation; we work *from* our salvation!

Jesus Christ was the runner who won the prize on our behalf! It is by God's grace and God's grace alone that we have been called to serve the true and living Lord. How does the fact that you are God's workmanship, His handcrafted creation, help you understand why participation in First Place 4 Health is part of your proper response to God's grace?

---
---
---

What have you learned from today's lesson about this race you are called to run?

---
---
---
---

*O gracious Lord, help me to never forget that I can only run the race because Jesus won the battle against evil and empowers me to run in His power. Amen.*

## Day 6 — REFLECTION AND APPLICATION

*Mighty and sovereign Lord, thank You for calling me to love and serve You, not for the reward I might receive, but for the privilege of sharing in Your joy. Amen.*

During our Day Four study, we read the Parable of the Talents, a teaching story Jesus told His disciples about the importance of prudently managing all that the Master has entrusted to our care. (If you would like to refresh your memory, turn to Matthew 25:14-30 in your Bible.) Yes, the parable has a second teaching we are not covering in this week's study—the fate of the unfaithful servant—but for this study, we are concentrating our efforts on what the parable teaches about being faithful and fruitful.

This parable is not just about money and investing our money in God's kingdom, although prudent financial management is part of the stewardship

God calls us to practice. This parable is about wisely managing *all* that God has entrusted to our care in a way that leads to an increase in God's kingdom.

If your Lord and Master were to return tonight for an accounting of the way you have managed the good gifts He has entrusted to you, what kind of report would you be able to give? As you answer this question, know that this is not about salvation. All who call on the name of Jesus will be saved. This parable is about accountability before God for the way we have managed all our affairs on His behalf. Begin your accounting with how you have cared for your physical body, which God Himself handcrafted according to His exact specifications. Then extend your account to include your spiritual gifts, your talents, your education and experience, your family—all the good things that God has blessed you with so that you can be a blessing to others. Write in your prayer journal for privacy.

After you finish your account, listen to your Lord and Master praise you for being faithful with a few things as a prelude to the additional things you will be given—and feel the joy of entering into your Master's happiness.

*My Lord and Master, thank You for Your marvelous grace and for allowing me to be Your faithful steward as I work to build Your kingdom here on Earth. Amen.*

## REFLECTION AND APPLICATION  Day 7

*Faithful Shepherd, thank You for calling me to be one of Your flock and for taking such good care of me. Amen.*

For the past two weeks we have been learning about Olympic-type runners competing to win the prize—faithful shepherds of the flock who will receive a crown of glory when the Chief Shepherd appears and faithful servants who managed the Master's affairs. Today we are going to exercise "stop and think about it" muscles as we reflect on what these analogies have taught us.

From comparing our faith journey to training for an Olympic race, what have you learned about living a life pleasing to God?

_____

_____

_____

_____

When will you receive the reward for your faithful service?

From the Parable of the Talents, what did you learn about the importance of wholehearted stewardship?

And, finally, what did you learn about God's grace and your ability to run the race and win the prize in your own strength and power?

How will all of these lessons help you to press on toward your First Place 4 Health goals?

*O Lord, I can only run the race because You empower me to run. I can only prudently manage the things You have entrusted to my care because You teach me about storing up treasures in heaven. I can only put one foot in front of the other because You are holding my hand. Amen.*

## *Group Prayer Requests*

4health first place

Today's Date: _____

| Name | Request |
|------|---------|
|      |         |
|      |         |
|      |         |
|      |         |
|      |         |
|      |         |
|      |         |
|      |         |
|      |         |
|      |         |

Results

_____

_____

_____

_____

_____

_____

_____

## Week Nine

# breaking free

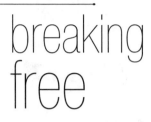

SCRIPTURE MEMORY VERSE

*Therefore, since we are surrounded by such a great cloud of witnesses, let us throw off everything that hinders and the sin that so easily entangles, and let us run with perseverance the race marked out for us.*

HEBREWS 12:1

Throughout our Bible study, we have looked at some of the basic principles of Scripture interpretation that give us the ability to handle God's Word like a worker approved by God Himself. Summarize what you have learned during this Bible study that will allow you to better understand the truth of Scripture.

How is being able to correctly understand God's Word essential to this lifelong First Place 4 Health journey you are undertaking?

Imagine for a moment that you are in a strange city, trying to find your way to a specific address. You have a roadmap to guide your journey, but somehow you still can't find exactly where it is you are supposed to be. Each road you take leads nowhere. Then, to your frustration, you discover the map you are reading is the map of a city different from the one you are presently in. That's what happens to us when we don't properly interpret God's Word. No matter how diligent our efforts, we can never quite find our way.

How are the diet and exercise programs you were in prior to joining First Place 4 Health like trying to find a specific address with a map of a city different from the one you are in?

## OUR CHEERING SECTION

*Merciful Father, thank You for including in the Bible the stories of the faithful saints who have gone before us. Their courage helps me in my weakness. Their example gives me a pattern to follow. Amen.*

One of the principles of Scripture interpretation we have discussed involves the word "therefore." What are we to do whenever we see a sentence that begins with the word "therefore"?

Hebrews 11 is like the Bible's Hall of Fame, except instead of pictures and memorabilia, this Hall of Fame is filled with stories about the faith in action that these courageous men and women displayed. We learned about one of the members of this Hall of Fame during our Week Three Bible study. Who was this Bible great, and what did he do that made his faith story significant?

How does Hebrews 11:6 describe faith that pleases God?

Do you really believe God will reward your efforts as you earnestly seek Him through participation in First Place 4 Health?

_____

_____

What might that reward look like? As you answer this question, remember the four aspects of your being: physical, mental, emotional and spiritual. Also remember what you learned about the reward Jesus told us we will receive when the Master returns.

_____

_____

All of the saints listed in Hebrews 11 have entered into their Master's happiness, yet they have not retired! They were faithful in a few things, and now they have been given more. Based on what our memory verse for this week tells us about them, what is part of their current assignment?

_____

_____

They are encouraging us, cheering us on, as we press on and tread in their faithful footsteps. Spend some time thanking God for giving us faith examples to follow so that we are not moving through uncharted territory as we move forward together in our faith.

> _You, O Lord, have given me everything I need to run the race set before me. I can step out in faith because I know You are with me every step of the way. Amen._

## Day 2 — HINDRANCES

_Compassionate Father, there are so many things in the world I live in that get in the way of the life I know You are calling me to live. Thank You for sending Jesus to show me the way. Amen._

Our Week Nine memory verse begins with the word "therefore" and contains two implied commands.

Write the memory verse, and then circle the "Let Us" commands.

_____

_____

_____

What do the words "let us" in this verse tell you about the author of the book of Hebrews?

_____

_____

_____

Although this unknown person was writing the letter to the Hebrew Christians, he or she also struggled with the hindrances and sins that keep us entangled! Will there ever be a time while we are still on this earth in bodily form that we will not have to throw off the things that hinder us and the sin that so easily entangles? Explain your answer using principles and beliefs we have learned during this Bible study.

_____

_____

_____

_____

In order to really comprehend what is being said in the first "Let Us" of this week's memory verse, it is important that we correctly understand the meaning of the word "hinder." Look up the word "hinder" in a dictionary and write the meanings you find.

_____

_____

_____

The things that hinder us are the *external* things that hold us back and interfere with or obstruct our action or progress; therefore, a hindrance is anything that impedes or obstructs progress. What are the external things that keep you from moving forward in the First Place 4 Health program? Remember, hindrances are not about inner attitudes or thoughts; they are about exterior things that stand in our path or hold us back. One example of a hindrance would be sugar- and fat-laden snack food in the kitchen cabinets. List at least five people, places or things that hinder you from moving forward.

_____

_____

_____

Our memory verse tells us to "throw off" the things that hinder. Beside each of the five hindrances you listed above, write one thing you can do to begin eliminating that obstacle. For instance, if sugar- and fat-laden snacks in the cupboard are one of your hindrances, you can remove those foods from your cabinets and throw them away. (You might want to write the "throw off" action in a different color ink so that it is easy to identify.)

_____

_____

_____

Before we end today's study, there is one more word we need to highlight. Go back to the memory verse you wrote out and underline the word "everything." Does the word "everything" allow for exceptions or excuses? Why or why not?

_____

_____

_____

_O Lord God Almighty, thank You for walking with me on this journey and helping me identify and eliminate the things that keep me from moving forward in Christ Jesus my Lord. Amen._

## Day 3 ENTANGLING SIN

_Thank You, loving Lord, for giving me brothers and sisters to move forward together with me and encourage me to do my personal best. Amen._

Unlike the external things that hinder our forward progress, "the sin that easily entangles" is our own personal weaknesses—things inside of us—our Achilles heel, so to speak. Like it or not, each of us has specific weaknesses, just as each of us has specific strengths. Stop for a moment and think about your own personal vulnerability when it comes to the First Place 4 Health program. Some of us are "closet eaters"; others go out with binge buddies when we overindulge. Some of us worry; others deny that they have a problem. Some of us stuff down anger with food; others of us spew our anger onto everything and everyone around us. What is the personal sin pattern that keeps you in doubt and despair?

_____

_____

_____

Why do you think it is important to identify our areas of vulnerability?

_____

_____

_____

Our memory verse says we are to throw off "the sin." Does this mean there is only one sin we need to throw off, or does "the sin" refer to the collective sins that make up the sin that keeps us entangled? Explain your answer.

_____

_____

_____

While we may have many sins that combine to become "the sin that so easily entangles," there is one root sin common to all humanity: doing things our way rather than God's way. Throughout Scripture we see God's people being hardheaded and rebellious as they go outside God's established boundaries in search of greener pastures. Hebrews 3:12-15 gives us both the diagnosis and the tonic for the sin that so easily entangles us. What is the problem and what is the antidote as described in Hebrews 3:12-15?

Problem: _____

_____

Antidote: _____

_____

How is continuing to eat food that does not promote health and habitually failing to exercise, even after we know the truth of the First Place 4 Health program, rebelling against God?

Hebrews 3:13 tells us we can be hardened by sin's deceitfulness. How can your First Place 4 Health group keep you from falling into denial? (The answer is found in the same verse.)

Does the phrase "one another" mean that one person in the group does all the encouraging and the others in the group are recipients of encouraging words, or does it imply mutual encouragement? Explain your answer.

Are you doing your part when it comes to encouraging the others in your First Place 4 Health group? Why or why not?

End today's lesson by writing a note of encouragement to someone in your group who is struggling to overcome hindrances and sin.

*Gracious God, it is so easy for me to pick and choose those portions of Your Word that I want to obey while overlooking commands like "Encourage one another." Forgive me for not supporting others as I want them to support me. Amen.*

## PERSEVERANCE Day 4

*O Lord God, it is so much easier to enjoy instant gratification than to persevere in my faith. Please give me strength to finish the course, not start out quickly but soon fade away. Amen.*

The second "Let Us" in this week's memory verse uses the running analogy again. What are we told to do, and how are we to do it?

Turn again to Luke 8:15, and after reading the verse, compare it to what is said in the second "Let Us" of this week's memory verse.

Does the word "perseverance" in our memory verse imply speed or endurance? Explain your answer.

Many diet and exercise programs on the market today offer "instant" results. How are these immediate-gratification and instant-transformation programs a hindrance to your First Place 4 Health endeavors?

As long as you keep thinking there must be an easier, quicker way to lose weight, will you persevere when the road gets difficult and progress is slow? Explain.

The word "persevere" means to maintain one's purpose in spite of difficulty, obstacles or discouragement; to continue steadfastly when faced with opposition. What is implied by our memory verse telling us to run with perseverance?

_____

_____

_____

According to John 16:33, Jesus confirmed that we would have obstacles in our lives, but why did Jesus say we are to take heart?

_____

_____

_____

While we think of obstacles as things that make the journey more difficult, Jesus' brother James explained their purpose differently. What does the Lord's brother tell us in James 1:2-4?

_____

_____

_____

What do trials (another word for "hindrances") develop, according to James 1:3?

_____

_____

_____

And what does perseverance result in? (James 1:4 has the answer.)

_____

_____

_____

If Christian maturity is our goal, how should we view those things that result in our being mature and complete?

_____

_____

_____

How might thankfulness in difficulty be a way of throwing off the things that hinder you? Explain your answer thoroughly!

_____

_____

_____

Spend the rest of your quiet time thanking God for the trials that have taught you to persevere in your faith.

> *O Lord, when I lean on my own understanding rather than trusting in You, I do not allow trials to contribute to my growth in grace and knowledge. Please forgive me for not trusting more completely in You. Amen.*

## THE RACE MARKED OUT FOR US

Day 5

*Gracious God, You are the One who marks out my course before me and steadies my feet as I run the race You have set before me. Amen.*

In our Week Seven study, our lessons focused on the specific example the apostle Paul used to explain how we were to run the race marked out before us. What analogy did Paul use?

_____

_____

_____

Most of us are familiar with the Olympic Games, which are now both summer and winter events. Is there just one competitive event, or are there many races and meets that comprise the Olympic Games?

_____

_____

_____

What determines which event(s) a particular athlete will compete in?

_____

_____

_____

Do all of the competition courses look the same? For instance, does a high hurdler face the same challenges as the high jumper, or does each event have its own specific course and require different skills, talents and training?

In Ephesians 4:1-14, the apostle Paul tells us that we each have been given special gifts. Read this passage prayerfully. Who, according to Ephesians 4:7, is the One who determines the gifts and talents we each receive?

What is the ultimate goal for all Christians, even though they have different spiritual gifts and talents? (Ephesians 4:12-13 has the answer.)

Earlier in this week's study, we acknowledged that we each have individual and specific sin patterns that easily entangle us. We each also have unique circumstances that hinder our progress, and we each have different life experiences and personal histories. So though we strive for the same goal, has God marked out the same course for all of us? Why or why not?

If we spend our time and energy comparing our progress with that of others in our First Place 4 Health group, will we have time and energy left to devote to the race God has given us? Why or why not?

Recall our Week Seven lesson. Who is it that we compete against: self or others?

Last week's memory verse came from 1 Peter 5. Near the very end of the passage we studied in last week's lessons, Peter tells us who will restore us and make us steadfast, strong and firm. Read 1 Peter 5:10, and identify that person.

What does 1 Peter 5:11 tell us about God?

How has God's might and power helped you run the race set before you in First Place 4 Health? Spend the rest of your quiet time today praising Him for all He has done for you!

> *O Lord God, You are the One who keeps me from falling. You steady my faltering steps and show me the race You would have me run. Amen.*

## REFLECTION AND APPLICATION

**Day 6**

> *O Lord, thank You for always making the lessons You know I need to learn specific to my situation and age-appropriate for my level of Christian maturity. Amen.*

Not only does our gracious God design our course and mark out the race before us, He also does so in a way that brings balance and wholeness to our disordered lives. While we may neglect one aspect of our being in favor of one or two others, God desires maturity, and maturity takes balance. Today, think of the lessons God has taught you through this Bible study—lessons that have been specifically designed by your Creator for each part of your being. The elements of the four-sided person are shown in the table on the next page. In each quadrant, write the lessons God has taught you in that area during this study.

| PHYSICAL | MENTAL |
|---|---|
| EMOTIONAL | SPIRITUAL |

Were your lessons balanced, or were they concentrated in one or two areas? Explain your answer.

_____

_____

_____

_____

_____

What does the way God is working in your life tell you about your need for balance and wholeness?

_____

_____

_____

_____

Spend some time thanking God for being your teacher, your personal trainer and your guide.

*Father God, You know me better than I know myself. Please continue to search me and show me where I need to add strength and balance so that I can live and move and have my being in You. Amen.*

## REFLECTION AND APPLICATION

*Lord, help me to resist the devil and draw near to You rather than draw near to temptation and resist Your grace. Amen.*

One of the spiritual principles we learned earlier in the Bible study is the principle of replacement. What is the principle of replacement, and how does it work to bring balance and wholeness?

_____

_____

Our Week Nine memory verse illustrates the principle of replacement, as does one other memory verse from our Bible study. Identify the other replacement principle memory verse, and then write out both verses. In each verse, circle the vice we are to eliminate, and underline the virtue we are told to cultivate in its place. (Hint: In the other verse [see Week Six if you have trouble remembering], what we are to eliminate is implied but not specifically named.)

_____

_____

_____

What is one thing you have eliminated from your behavior or belief system as a result of this Bible study, and what did you replace it with?

_____

_____

Is the replacement principle a one-time practice, or a lifestyle?

_____

_____

*Gracious God, You call me to be holy and set apart. I can only be obedient to that command when I am willing to eliminate the things that keep me from running the race with perseverance. Forgive me when I fail to do so. Amen.*

## *Group Prayer Requests*

4 first place
health

Today's Date: _____

| Name | Request |
|------|---------|
|      |         |
|      |         |
|      |         |
|      |         |
|      |         |
|      |         |
|      |         |
|      |         |
|      |         |
|      |         |

Results

_____
_____
_____
_____
_____
_____

# focused
# on the prize

SCRIPTURE MEMORY VERSE

*Let us fix our eyes on Jesus, the author and perfecter of our faith, who for the joy set before him endured the cross, scorning its shame, and sat down at the right hand of the throne of God.*

HEBREWS 12:2

At the beginning of His earthly ministry, Jesus of Nazareth went into the synagogue on the Sabbath, as was His custom. And when Jesus, the living Word, stood up to read from the written Word, He selected a passage from the prophecy of Isaiah: "The Spirit of the Lord is on me, because He has anointed me to preach good news to the poor. He has sent me to proclaim freedom for the prisoners and recovery of sight for the blind, to release the oppressed, to proclaim the year of the Lord's favor" (Luke 4:18-19; see also Isaiah 61:1-2). Luke goes on to tell us that after Jesus finished reading those powerful words, "the eyes of everyone in the synagogue were fastened on him" and Jesus told them, "Today this scripture is fulfilled in your hearing" (Luke 4:20-21).

As you read the words Jesus quoted that day in the synagogue, underline the specific things the Lord had anointed Jesus to do while He was here on Earth. How might the First Place 4 Health program be an anointed extension of Jesus' earthly ministry? How are people hearing the good news, receiving spiritual sight, being set free from the things that keep them spiritually oppressed, and learning to walk in God's favor as they participate in First Place 4 Health?

_____

_____

_____

_____

As you contemplate the things Jesus came to Earth to do, think about the things you need most in your life right now. Reread Luke 4:18-19. Allow the Spirit of the living Lord to show you what God has anointed Jesus to do for you. Do you need to hear the good news, receive spiritual sight, be set free from bondage and spiritual oppression, or learn to walk in God's favor? As you think about the things you need today, ask Jesus of Nazareth to come into the synagogue of your heart, bringing hope and healing.

## Day 1 EYES THAT SEE

*O Lord God, You will keep me in perfect peace*
*when my eyes are focused on You. Amen.*

Our memory verse for Week Ten is an extension of the memory verse we learned last week: another "Let Us" command. What were the two "Let Us" commands we learned about through last week's study?

_____

_____

When we combine last week's memory verse with this week's verse, we have a great example of the principle of replacement. Write out the two verses together (this week's verse and Hebrews 12:1-2). After you have completed writing, draw a line through the things we are to throw off and circle the things we are to replace them with.

_____

_____

_____

What have you done since last week's Bible study to weed out those things that keep you mired in destructive habits?

_____

_____

_____

What new behaviors—life-giving practices—have you put into place to replace destructive habits?

_____

_____

_____

Our memory verse for this week tells us to do something specific with our eyes. What are we to do, and why are we to do it?

_____

_____

_____

As we saw in the introduction to this week's study, one of the things Jesus came to give was sight to the blind. And although Jesus did physically heal those who could not see during His earthly ministry, His primary purpose was to give us another type of sight. What type of sight did Jesus come to give? (Ephesians 1:18 has the answer, so read that verse before answering this question.)

_____

_____

_____

How have the eyes of your heart been enlightened as you have completed the daily lessons in _Moving Forward Together_?

_____

_____

_____

When Jesus encountered Bartimaeus beside the road leading to Jericho, the blind beggar had one request of Jesus. Turn to Mark 10:51 and read both Jesus' question and Bartimaeus's reply. Now imagine Jesus is standing before you right now asking the same thing: "What do you want Me to do for you?" What type of sight do you need to ask the miracle-working Jesus to give you?

_____

_____

_____

Spend the remainder of your quiet time asking Jesus to open the eyes of your heart so that you can see Him more clearly. Read Mark 10:51 at the end of your time with the Lord, and leave your quiet place confident that your faith has restored your inner sight so that you can follow Jesus with a new vision.

*O Lord, You and You alone can open the inner eyes of my heart. For so long I walked in darkness. Thank You for sending Jesus to show me the way and for giving me the inner vision to follow Him. Amen.*

Day
2

## FOCUS ON JESUS

*Open my eyes, Lord, that I may see the marvelous truths contained in Your Word. Thank You, Lord. Amen.*

Recorded in the Gospels are many incidents of Jesus' healing blind people, yet one particular account has some valuable lessons to teach those of us who grope in spiritual blindness when it comes to caring for ourselves. Turn to John 9:1-3 in your Bible and prayerfully read these verses. What is the first thing John 9:1 tells us?

_____

_____

Even though the man was blind, Jesus was not, and He noticed the blind man. What hope does that wonderful truth give you?

_____

_____

_____

When you were stumbling along in darkness with regard to caring for ourselves, what did Jesus see and do?

_____

_____

_____

Before Jesus began to interact with the blind man, His disciples asked Him a question. What was that question?

_____

_____

_____

How is this question applicable to those who are trapped in the bondage of out-of-control eating?

_____

_____

_____

Poor eating and exercise patterns are both familial and generational. How have the eating and exercise habits you learned in your family of origin been part of your struggle?

_____

_____

_____

Jesus did not want the disciples to focus their attention on whom to blame for the problem that exists. What did Jesus say to the disciples to give them a new perspective? (John 9:3 has the answer.)

_____

_____

_____

Rather than focusing on the man's sins or the sins of his parents, Jesus invited His disciples to contemplate God's might and power. How can Jesus' words help you refocus your energy—especially the energy you have spent on blaming others for your problems rather than keeping your eyes on the Source of your healing?

_____

_____

_____

How can your out-of-control eating be used so that the work of God might be displayed in your life as you receive inner sight through First Place 4 Health?

_____

_____

Where is your focus to be as we move forward together: on the problem or on Jesus (the solution)? What is one thing you can do today to keep your eyes focused on Jesus?

_____

_____

_____

*Thank You, Lord, for allowing me to look to Jesus for inner strength rather than blame others for the problems that brought me to First Place 4 Health. Amen.*

## Day 3 — LOOK AND BE HEALED

*Lord, so often I grow impatient and fail to wait for Your timing. Help me to persevere along the journey and be thankful for Your many blessings. Amen.*

Long before Jesus, the living Word of God, came to live among us in human form, God gave His people many signs and symbols that foretold what the ministry of Jesus would accomplish while He was here on Earth. One of those symbols was a bronze snake Moses was commanded to put on a pole. Turn to Numbers 21:4-9 in your Bible and read this account.

The Israelites were in the desert, making the long, arduous journey from the bondage of Egypt to the freedom of the land God had promised them. Earlier in our Bible study, we learned about that promise. Who was it first given to, and how did the man who first received the promise respond? (This was the subject of our Week Three Bible study.)

_____

_____

But Numbers 21:4 tells us that something happened to the people making the journey. What happened?

_____

_____

_____

How is growing impatient on the way different from the perseverance we studied in last week's lessons?

_____

_____

_____

In their impatience, God's Chosen People said something that is all too familiar to most of us in First Place 4 Health. What did the people say? Rephrase the words given in Numbers 21:5 to reflect how you have probably felt at times during your First Place 4 Health journey.

_____

_____

_____

The people grumbled and complained because there was no bread and no water. What type of "bread" have you missed during this journey, even though you had all the nourishing manna you needed to sustain life and promote health? And what grumbling words have you said about the food on the Live It Plan? Be honest with your answer.

_____

_____

_____

Because of the people's grumbling and complaining, the Lord sent venomous snakes to inflict them. What types of venomous snakes are always our traveling companions when we grumble and complain rather than thank God for His faithful provision for all of our needs?

_____

_____

_____

In their distress, the people came to Moses and asked that he pray for them. What does Numbers 21:7 tell us the people said to Moses?

How is this like the confession we learned about in our Week Five study?

In response to the people's cries for help, God gave Moses some instructions. Read Numbers 21:8 and write down what the Lord said to Moses. After you have written down God's words, underline the portion that foreshadows the truth given in this week's memory verse.

Moses did as God commanded, and Numbers 21:9 tells us that the people who looked at the snake that was put up on the pole lived. Jesus referred to this incident in the desert when describing His mission and ministry. Turn to John 3:14-15. What did Jesus say about the snake Moses lifted up in the desert?

Look back at the grumbling and complaining you have done along the journey. How can looking to Jesus, the author and perfecter of your faith, take the sting out of the fiery serpents that keep you from enjoying God's presence and love?

What does this lesson teach us about the importance of knowing God's salvation story as it is recorded in both the Old and New Testaments?

_____

_____

_____

_____

*O Lord God, today I will turn my eyes upon Jesus, knowing that as I look at His face, the troubles of this life will pale in comparison to His radiance. Amen.*

## LOOKING DOWN

**Day 4**

*Wonderful Savior, You see me long before I see You, and You bring Your healing touch to the things that keep me from moving forward. Amen.*

Although Jesus physically healed the blind during His earthly ministry, He also brought healing to those who could not look at Him because of other infirmities. Luke 13:10-17 gives us an account of a woman who could not see Jesus, not because her eyes were blind, but because her back was bent. Read her story now and make note of the thing that kept her bound.

_____

_____

_____

Again, it was the Sabbath, and Jesus was in a synagogue. Recall from the introduction to this week's study why Jesus went to the synagogue on the Sabbath.

_____

_____

_____

Is it also your custom to go to church on the Sabbath? Why or why not?

_____

_____

_____

The woman in today's Gospel story also went to the synagogue on the Sabbath, even though she was crippled by a spirit that kept her bent over. What does this tell you about spiritual maladies that impact people who make it their custom to attend public worship?

It is also important to note that although Satan had kept this woman bound for 18 long years (Luke 13:16 gives us that fact), she was not demon possessed. Why is it important that we make a distinction between being crippled by a spirit and possessed by a demon?

Jesus did not need to cast a demon from this woman as He had done for those who were demon possessed; all Jesus needed to do was release her from the spirit that kept her bound. What spirit that keeps you bound in destructive self-care habits does Jesus need to release you from today?

Picture this poor woman's physical condition in your mind. Luke, the physician, gives us a very graphic picture of her infirmity. What does Luke 13:11 tell us about her?

This is not an occasional bout of sciatica. The woman was totally bent over and unable to look at anything but the ground. Given her physical condition, could this woman see Jesus as He stood at the front of the synagogue?

But Jesus saw her! How does this correspond to what we learned about the blind man in our Day Two lesson?

When Jesus saw the woman and realized the extent of her malady, what did Jesus do, and how did the woman respond? (See Luke 13:12 for the answer.)

Not only did Jesus call her forward, He also did something else. What else did Jesus do? (The answer is in Luke 13:13.)

What happened when Jesus put His hands on this woman?

How is Jesus touching and healing you from the spirit that keeps you bent over and unable to fix your eyes on Him?

Spend the rest of your quiet time today praising God for the wonderful things He is doing for you in the First Place 4 Health program.

*O Lord, when I was lost, You saw me. When I was in distress, You cured me. Thank You for seeing my plight and coming to my rescue. Amen.*

# FOCUSED ON THE SOLUTION, NOT THE PROBLEM

*Lord God, You know that I am often distracted by the problems that those close to me are having, and rather than look to You, I focus on their situation. Help me to bring those I love and care for to You, in faith that You care for them—and for me. Amen.*

In the Gospel of Mark, we see another situation that can keep us from fixing our eyes on Jesus: the care and concern we have for those we love. Turn to Mark 9:17-27, and read about this event, an event that occurred right after Jesus came down from the mountain on which the Transfiguration had taken place. After reading this story, summarize what happened in your own words, as if you were an on-the-spot reporter speaking to a television audience.

-------------------------------------------------------------------------

-------------------------------------------------------------------------

-------------------------------------------------------------------------

-------------------------------------------------------------------------

How is the way Jesus ministered to this demon-possessed boy different from the way He healed the blind man in our Day Two lesson and the crippled woman we learned about yesterday?

-------------------------------------------------------------------------

-------------------------------------------------------------------------

-------------------------------------------------------------------------

What does this tell you about Jesus' ability to correctly diagnose and properly treat the things that keep us from fixing our eyes on Him?

-------------------------------------------------------------------------

-------------------------------------------------------------------------

-------------------------------------------------------------------------

Mark tells us what the boy's physical symptoms were, much like Luke described the crippled woman for us in yesterday's lesson. How did the evil spirit manifest itself in the young boy's life (Mark 9:17-18)?

-------------------------------------------------------------------------

-------------------------------------------------------------------------

-------------------------------------------------------------------------

The spirit was causing the helpless boy to do many destructive things. Think of someone in your life who is on a self-destructive path right now, a person whose problems dim your vision of Jesus, and write the details of the situation.

What did Jesus command the concerned father to do (Mark 9:19)?

Jesus asked the boy's father to tell Him about the problem in more detail. What did the father say to Jesus in Mark 9:21-22? Please pay particular attention to the word "if" at the beginning of the last sentence in verse 22.

How did Jesus respond to the concerned parent (Mark 9:23)?

Rather than focus on the problem, what did Jesus ask the worried father to do?

How is having faith like keeping our eyes fixed on Jesus, even when those we love and care about are out of control?

In response to the father's faith statement, Jesus commanded the spirit to come out of the boy. Pay careful attention to what happened next. What does Mark 9:26 tell us happened when Jesus commanded the spirit to leave the boy?

_____

_____

_____

_____

Yes, often the problem seems to get worse before it gets better. When challenged by God's truth, Satan always puts up a fight! It would have been easy for those in the crowd that day to look at what the spirit had done to the boy rather than believe Jesus was the Great Physician. What does Mark 9:26 tell us many of the people in the crowd said?

_____

_____

_____

Did Jesus believe the same thing? What did Jesus do (Mark 9:27)?

_____

_____

_____

What worry or concern about those you love and care for is keeping you from running the course set out before you in First Place 4 Health, and if Jesus were here today, what would He ask you to do? (Our memory verse and today's lesson have the answer.)

_____

_____

_____

_____

*O Lord God, thank You for showing me how to deal with the cares and concerns that burden my heart when those I love and care about are careening out of control. Help me, gracious Lord, to keep my eyes on You and have faith that You will bring about healing in Your perfect time and Your perfect way. Amen.*

## REFLECTION AND APPLICATION

*My Lord and my God, You are the solution, no matter what the problem.*
*Help me to keep my eyes focused on You and not on the things of this world*
*that distract and disturb me. You came, Lord Jesus, to give me peace. Amen.*

Yesterday we read the account of the young boy whose father brought him to
Jesus, the Divine Physician. Summarize what you learned from that lesson that
will help you move forward in faith rather than be bogged down with doubt
and fear.

Although we stopped our study yesterday at Mark 9:27, there is an important
lesson to be learned from Mark 9:28-29. Read those verses now and record
what Jesus said.

Although the *NIV* translates Jesus' words as "This kind can come out only by
prayer," other Bible translations add the word "fasting": "This kind can come
out only by prayer and fasting" (*KJV*). How are prayer and "fasting" (which is
not limited to abstaining from food but also may include any form of refrain-
ing from whatever it is that keeps us from focusing our eyes on God) part of
the First Place 4 Health program?

With that knowledge, how can you use prayer and "fasting" as your spiritual
worship of God, worship that is a physical manifestation of your faith statement that everything is possible for those who believe in Jesus?

Make a list of those you will bring before Jesus in prayer and fasting, confident that He will touch and heal them in wonderful ways.

_____

_____

_____

_____

*O gracious Lord, all too often I forget that prayer and fasting are time-honored disciplines that bring me into Your presence in a powerful way. Help me to realize that when I humble myself before You, You lift up me and those I care about. Amen.*

## Day 7 REFLECTION AND APPLICATION

*O Lord, You have done wonderful things for me, and I am filled with joy! Amen.*

During this week's lessons, we have looked at the marvelous ways Jesus, the Divine Physician, touched and healed those suffering from diseases that kept them from fixing their eyes on Him. Our lessons this week have shown us examples of three different people Jesus healed. Who were those three people, and what did Jesus do for them? In your recap, include how each healing story is similar to the other two, and how each story is different and unique to the needs of the suffering individual.

_____

_____

_____

_____

Next week we will conclude our Bible study. As part of the victory celebration on Week Twelve, you will be asked to talk about the wonderful things God has done for you during this First Place 4 Health session. Using the stories of the three people Jesus healed, along with the account of the serpent being lifted up in the desert, and our replacement-principle studies, begin writing your story by praising God for the unique way He has touched and healed you during this First Place 4 Health session.

*Gracious God, what a privilege it is to recount the wonderful things You have done for me! Prepare the hearts and minds of those who will hear my words so that they will receive new insight from the marvelous things You have done. Amen.*

## *Group Prayer Requests*

4 first place health

Today's Date: _____

| Name | Request |
|------|---------|
|  |  |
|  |  |
|  |  |
|  |  |
|  |  |
|  |  |
|  |  |
|  |  |
|  |  |
|  |  |

Results

_____

_____

_____

_____

_____

_____

_____

# Week Eleven

# binding it
# all together

SCRIPTURE MEMORY VERSE
*See to it that no one misses the grace of God and that
no bitter root grows up to cause trouble and defile many.*
HEBREWS 12:15

Our Scripture memory verses for Weeks Nine and Ten also came from Hebrews 12, the chapter in which this week's memory verse appears. Both verses contained the command "Let us." What were the three "Let Us" statements in the memory verses for Weeks Nine and Ten?

Let us _____ .

Let us _____ .

Let us _____ .

But in our Scripture memory verse for Week Eleven we see a different command at the beginning of the verse. What is that little three-word command?

_____   _____   _____

Why do you think the writer of the book of Hebrews is no longer including him- or herself in the statement?

_____

_____

_____

_____

Yes, the writer is already seeing to it that no one misses the grace of God! He or she crafted this wonderful epistle to prove that Jesus Christ is the spotless Lamb of God, the One sent to be the once-and-for-all sacrifice that makes us right with God. But in addition to telling us to see to it that no one misses the grace of God, the author of Hebrews asks us to do one more thing according to this week's memory verse. What is the second part of the exhortation contained in Hebrews 12:15?

_____

_____

_____

What do these words tell us about how bitterness can impact even those who have been saved by God's grace?

_____

_____

_____

## NOXIOUS WEEDS AND BITTER ROOTS

Day 1

*O Lord God, when I keep my eyes on You, I will not fall prey to the things that have the ability to keep me from being Your faithful and fruitful servant. Amen.*

During our Week Four Bible study, we learned about some noxious weeds that had the potential to choke out the good plants before they had an opportunity to bear fruit. Write the Week Four memory verse, and underline three things we are to eliminate before they hinder our ability to move forward.

_____

_____

_____

Can you see a connection between the weeds that have the ability to keep the growing plants from producing a crop and the bitter root that has the potential to cause trouble and defile? In giving your answer, remember that the growing plants came from seeds that fell on good ground. Unlike the seeds that fell by the path and the ones that landed in rocky ground, these seeds were able to produce a crop; they had received the grace of God!

Those of us who have gardened know that weeds cannot simply be whacked off at ground level. What do we need to do in order to eradicate the weeds?

How could a root of bitterness produce worries of this life, deceitfulness of wealth and a desire for other things? Remember that bitterness comes from thinking we have been treated unjustly and haven't gotten our fair share.

What did our Week Six memory verse instruct us to do when dealing with those things that could defile us?

How can a bitter root cause trouble for you as you move forward toward your health and wholeness goals in the First Place 4 Health program? And what can you pursue instead of succumbing to the toxic poison of a bitter root?

*O gracious and loving God, You call me to be holy, because You are holy and I bear Your likeness through the new life given to me in Jesus Christ my Lord. Amen.*

## THE SOURCE OF BITTERNESS

*O merciful Father, help me to understand my part in the bitterness*
*that has the potential to hinder my First Place 4 Health progress. Amen.*

As part of our Week Ten Bible study lessons, we read about an incident that occurred while the Israelites were making the journey from the bondage of Egypt to the freedom of the Promised Land. Recap what you learned from the Day Three lesson in Week Ten.

_____

_____

_____

_____

Another desert story will help us better understand the root cause of bitterness. Turn to Exodus 15:22-25 in your Bible, and after reading this account, tell the story in your own words, as if you were reporting the events of the desert journey to an audience.

_____

_____

_____

_____

Just three days after witnessing the Lord's mighty act of parting the Red Sea so that the people could cross on dry ground, they started to grumble and complain. What was the cause of their displeasure? (Exodus 15:23 has the answer.)

_____

_____

_____

Why do you think the people grumbled and complained rather than ask Moses to pray for water? After all, they had just witnessed God's might and power three days before!

_____

_____

_____

Why do you grumble and complain instead of cry out to God for relief? After all, we witness the Lord's mighty acts on a daily basis as we move forward together in First Place 4 Health!

Exodus 15:25 tells us that Moses cried out to the Lord. How did God respond?

What happened when Moses threw the piece of wood into the water?

In the account of the venomous snakes, which also occurred because God's people grumbled and complained, what did the bronze snake on the pole symbolize? (You can reread the account in Numbers 21:4-9 if you need to refresh your memory.)

What do you think the piece of wood Moses was told to throw into the bitter water might symbolize?

How does the cross of Jesus Christ turn our bitter lives into sweetness?

Jesus can also take away the bitterness that threatens to cause you trouble. What do you need to do before Jesus can turn your bitterness into rejoicing?

_____

_____

_____

How is allowing Jesus to take away the bitterness of your life part of the First Place 4 Health program?

_____

_____

_____

*O Lord God, please forgive me for the times I grumble and complain rather than cry out to You in confidence that You will see, hear and come to my rescue. Amen.*

## THE SOURCE OF GRACE

**Day 3**

*O Lord, it is so easy to become discouraged and doubt Your promises, especially after years of cruel bondage to a destructive relationship with food. Amen.*

So far during our Bible study, we have studied two stories about the ancient Israelites during their desert wilderness experience. Where had God's people come from, and where were they going?

_____

_____

_____

Exodus 6:6-8 records the promises God made to the children of Israel before Moses led them out of captivity. What did God covenant to do for the people, and how was this a confirmation of the covenant God made with Abraham centuries before?

_____

_____

_____

Moses presented God's liberation plan to the Israelites, but they did not believe him. Why did the people not believe Moses? (Read Exodus 6:9 for the answer.)

_____

_____

_____

How has your discouragement and cruel bondage to a destructive relationship with food kept you from hearing God's Word?

_____

_____

_____

What did Abraham (discussed in our Week Three lessons) do when he became discouraged and doubted that God's promises to him could possibly come to pass? Use the words of our Week Two memory verse in your explanation of what Abraham did when discouraged.

_____

_____

_____

Abraham kept pressing on, even when he didn't know where he was going and didn't understand how God's promise of descendants more numerous than the stars in the sky could possibly come true. How have you been able to press on during this Bible study, even though you didn't understand how God's promise of restoration and vibrant health could be yours?

_____

_____

_____

Who is the One who has called you to make this journey to the Promised Land, and who is the One who walks with you every step of the way?

_____

_____

_____

God's promises are always "Yes" and "Amen." What our sovereign, supreme and all-powerful Lord plans and purposes will come to pass. What is your responsibility, your appropriate response to the grace shown you in Christ Jesus your Lord?

_____

_____

_____

Are you doing your part as you move forward with God toward the reward that awaits you when you enter into your Master's happiness? Why or why not?

_____

_____

_____

*O Lord God, You are faithful, and You are true to Your promises. Help me to do my part by stepping out in faith and doing all that You ask me to do along the way. Thank You. Amen.*

## THE FREEDOM OF FORGIVENESS

Day 4

*Jesus, You are the Lamb of God. You took all my sins, everything I will ever do wrong, and put them to death by nailing them to Calvary's cross. How can I ever express my gratitude for the gift of forgiveness? All I can do is live for You because You died for me. Amen.*

This week's memory verse asks that we "see to it that no one misses the grace of God and that no _____ _____ grows up to cause _____ and _____ many." During this week's study, what have you learned about the potential that a bitter root has to defile us?

_____

_____

_____

In our Day Two lesson, we learned that looking at a snake on a wooden pole cured people bitten by venomous snakes and that a piece of wood thrown into a pool of bitter water turned the water sweet. We also learned that both of these events were symbolic of Jesus' dying on a wooden cross. Why did Jesus suffer and die on Calvary's cross? (Isaiah 53:4-6 has the answer.)

Jesus took on all our sins—everything we have ever done wrong and everything we will ever do wrong—and put them to death when He died so that we could be forgiven. Read Paul's words in Romans 6:23. What did we deserve and what did we get instead?

Earlier in this week's study, we determined that bitterness is the result of feeling as if we have been treated unjustly, that we have not received our fair share—that our life has been difficult while others have been given an easier path to travel. And, yes, some of us have had cruel things happen to us. Often, memories of abuse are the bitter root that causes us to struggle with excess weight and out-of-control eating. How does Jesus' presence in the bitter water we have been given to drink transform our bitterness into a fountain of life?

Our Week Five memory verse came from Colossians 3:14. Write the verse below.

As you will recall, in order to understand what all these virtues were, we needed to go back five verses. Today we will just look at one of the virtues we are to put on. Turn to Colossians 3:13. What does that verse tell us to do?

How does forgiving whatever grievances we have against others deal with the root of bitterness?

According to Colossians 3:13, why do we forgive?

Just because we forgive others does not mean they will not be held accountable. Read Romans 12:17-19. What do we do when we let go of our need for revenge by forgiving those who have harmed us?

How does allowing God to be the One who deals with those who have harmed us free us to travel forward rather than being mired in the bitterness that keeps us stuck in the past?

If you were to forgive all the people who have ever harmed you, how would your participation in the First Place 4 Health program be different?

*O Lord, it is difficult to leave vengeance to You, especially when the hurt done to me in the past has lasting consequences. Yet I know that until I allow You to be the One who rights the wrongs done to me, I cannot move forward in faith. Amen.*

Day
5

# THE SWEETNESS OF REJOICING

*Father God, I have reason to rejoice because You have promised to never leave me or forsake me; You are always near. Amen.*

Recall from our earlier studies what it was the Israelites did when they encountered difficulty while on their journey from bondage to freedom.

_____

_____

Exodus 17 records another time when God's people grumbled and complained, except this time we are given more information about what they actually said. Turn to Exodus 17:7. What did people question?

_____

_____

How often is your grumbling and complaining the result of forgetting (or questioning) that the Lord has promised to always be with you, to never leave you or forsake you? Explain your answer.

_____

_____

Paul, in Philippians 4:4-7, gives us the universal antidote to grumbling and complaining. Read aloud Paul's words. Paul tells us to _____ . And lest we fail to hear his first statement, what does Paul do (Philippians 4:4)?

_____

_____

Philippians 4:5 tells us to let our gentleness be known to all. Which of our memory verses from the Bible study uses the word "gentleness"? Write that verse.

_____

_____

But Paul doesn't just tell us to let our gentleness be known to all; he also tells us how we can let this happen. What does Paul say in the last sentence of Philippians 4:5?

We can be gentle because the Lord is near. How is giving vengeance to God (from yesterday's Bible study lesson) something we must do before we can be gentle?

In Philippians 4:6, Paul tells us, "Do not be _____ about anything, but in _____ , by prayer and petition, with _____ , present your requests to God." What did our Week Four memory verse teach us about being anxious (or worrying)?

What does Philippians 4:6 tell us we are to replace our worry with?

As we pray, do we just rattle off our petitions, or is there another ingredient we are to add to our prayers, according to Philippians 4:6?

What happens when we present our prayers and petitions to God with thanksgiving? (Philippians 4:7 gives us the answer.)

How is having the peace of God guard our hearts and minds in Christ Jesus different from grumbling, complaining and questioning God's presence?

_____

_____

Using the principle of replacement we have learned during this Bible study, what can we replace bitterness with that will produce rejoicing?

_____

_____

How has this Bible study given you reason to rejoice because you are confident that the Lord is near and sees your needs before you are even aware that they exist?

_____

_____

*How grateful I am, loving Lord, that I can let my gentleness be known to all because You have taken away my bitterness. As a forgiven sinner, I know You are always with me to bless me. I can rejoice because You are always near. Amen.*

## Day 6 — REFLECTION AND APPLICATION

*Thank You, gracious God, that I can cast my cares on You and replace my disappointment and bitterness with joy as I draw close to You.*

Today, take a thankfulness walk! As you experience God's creation, meditate on your blessings. Sometimes when we have been hurt or disappointed, it's difficult to shift our focus to the good things in our life. But as you breathe the fresh air and notice the intricacy of our Creator's handiwork, thank Him for creating you with even greater care than the fragrant flower you stop to smell or the sun warming your back. Thank Him for the people He has brought into your life who love and support you. Consider gathering a few items from your walk that will remind you to count your blessings on a regular basis. Perhaps an acorn will bring your children to mind, or a small rock will remind you of your church. Be creative!

## REFLECTION AND APPLICATION

*You are the God of hope, the One who fills me with peace and joy
as I trust in You. Thank You for being the light of my life. Amen.*

All too soon, this session of First Place 4 Health is coming to an end! We have covered a lot of territory in our time together, and now we are planning to celebrate the victory we have in Jesus our Lord. During this time of joyous celebration, you will have an opportunity to briefly share the highlights of your *Moving Forward Together* journey with the others in your First Place 4 Health group.

Next week, rather than day-to-day Bible study, you'll find daily reflection questions that will help you write your testimony for the victory celebration at your group's Week Twelve meeting. As you write the summary of your journey in your spiritual journal, also review the memory verses and lessons we have covered during this study. You need not list them all, but include the major lessons you have learned through this 12-week session.

This is also the time for you to begin planning for the next leg of this life-long journey we are making toward health, restoration and a balanced lifestyle that pleases God. All of the First Place 4 Health Bible studies have been designed to give you strength and courage as you make this pilgrimage. Your group may have already selected the First Place 4 Health Bible study they will utilize during the next session. If not, please look over the list of Bible studies and help your group select the study that most closely fits your group's needs.

You might want to end your record of this First Place 4 Health session by committing to another session now. That way you can include your future hopes and dreams for health and wholeness at the conclusion of your testimony.

May God bless you richly as you write down words that will encourage and strengthen others—and add to your personal testimony that gives Jesus Christ first place in your life.

*Thank You, Lord, for allowing me to make this First Place 4 Health journey. Even now I commit my future plans to You, knowing that as I walk in Your will and way, my plans will succeed. Amen.*

## *Group Prayer Requests*

first place
4health

Today's Date: _____

| Name | Request |
|------|---------|
|  |  |
|  |  |
|  |  |
|  |  |
|  |  |
|  |  |
|  |  |
|  |  |
|  |  |
|  |  |

Results

_____

_____

_____

_____

_____

_____

*Week Twelve*

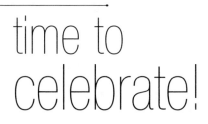

time to
celebrate!

To help you shape your brief victory celebration testimony, prayerfully work through the following questions in your spiritual journal, one on each day leading up to your group's celebration:

**Day One:** List some of the benefits you have gained by allowing the Lord to transform your life through this 12-week First Place 4 Health session. Be sure to list benefits you have received in the physical, mental, emotional and spiritual realms of your being

**Day Two:** In what ways have you most significantly changed *mentally*? Have you seen a shift in the ways you think about yourself, food, your relationships or God? How has Scripture memory been a part of these shifts?

**Day Three:** In what ways have you most significantly changed *emotionally*? Have you begun to identify how your feelings influence your relationship to food and exercise? What are you doing to stay aware of your emotions, both positive and negative?

**Day Four:** In what ways have you most significantly changed *spiritually*? How has your relationship with God deepened? How has drawing closer to Him made a difference in the other three areas of your life?

**Day Five:** In what ways have you most significantly changed *physically*? Have you met or exceeded your weight/measurement goals? How has your health improved during the past 12 weeks?

**Day Six:** Was there one person in your First Place 4 Health group who was particularly encouraging to you? How did their kindness make a difference in your First Place 4 Health journey?

**Day Seven:** Summarize the previous six questions into a one-page testimony, or "faith story," to share at your group's victory celebration.

May our gracious Lord bless and keep you as you continue to keep Him first in all things!

# *Moving Forward Together*
# leader discussion guide

For in-depth information, guidance and helpful tips about leading a successful First Place 4 Health group, spend time studying the *First Place 4 Health Leader's Guide*. In it, you will find valuable answers to most of your questions, as well as personal insights from many First Place 4 Health group leaders.

For the group meetings in this session, be sure to read and consider each week's discussion topics several days before the meeting—some questions and activities require supplies and/or planning to complete. Also, if you are leading a large group, plan to break into smaller groups for discussion and then come together as a large group to share your answers and responses. Make sure to appoint a capable leader for each small group so that discussions stay focused and on track (and be sure each group records their answers!).

## week one: welcome to *Moving Forward Together*

During this first week, welcome the members to your group, provide a brief overview of the First Place 4 Health program, explain what is expected of the participants at each of the weekly meetings, and collect the Member Surveys. (See the *First Place 4 Health Leader's Guide* for a detailed outline of how to conduct the first week's meeting.)

## week two: step by step

As you begin this new session of First Place 4 Health, it is important that you emphasize that First Place 4 Health is not a quick-fix, instant-results program. Begin today's session by talking about the difference between a quick trip and a lifelong journey.

Participants were asked to look up the verb "press" in a dictionary. Talk about the different definitions they found and how they all apply to the First Place 4 Health program.

In order to know what we are pressing on toward, it is important to define what the prize looks like! Put the words "physically," "mentally," "emotionally" and "spiritually" on a whiteboard or flip chart. Ask your group to talk about their goals in each of the four aspects of their being.

To illustrate "steady and even pressure," push against an object with uneven pressure. You can either press with both hands, or ask someone from your group to push with all their strength on one side while you barely exert any pressure. Discuss the outcome with your group.

During the Day Three study, we looked at the fruit we are to bear in First Place 4 Health. Lead a discussion about the fruit that will last in each of the four areas of our being.

In Philippians 3:12, Paul employs a marvelous play on words when he talks about taking hold of that for which Christ took hold of him. Ask your group what Christ took hold of them for. Record their answers on a whiteboard or flip chart. Be sure the group's answers stay focused on health and fitness issues.

According to 2 Samuel 24:24, David said he would not offer a sacrifice that cost him nothing. Talk about the cost of participation in First Place 4 Health, a cost that is not related to the small price of the Bible study book!

Find a maze puzzle in a magazine or Sunday School lesson book. Provide a copy to each participant and ask them to begin at the end and trace backward. Talk about how this is easier than starting at the beginning, and why.

We can only press on toward the prize when we are in Christ Jesus. Make sure that all your group members have an opportunity to accept Jesus as their Lord and Savior, if they have not previously done so. Those who made a profession years ago but have not practiced the words they professed might like to recommit their lives to Christ at this time.

## week three: stepping forward in faith

As you begin today's meeting, lead a discussion about the goals we have in First Place 4 Health; and discuss the fact that although we set these goals, we don't really know what they will look like when we finally get to our destination.

Ask your group to identify the two things we must believe when we come to God in faith (from Hebrews 11:6) and how believing those two things is an essential part of participation in First Place 4 Health.

Abram was asked to leave his homeland and his father's household and begin an unknown journey. Talk to your group about the things they may need to leave behind in order to make the First Place 4 Health journey. Record their answers on your flip chart or whiteboard.

Believing God's promises is difficult when in our own human thinking we don't see how they can possibly happen. Ask your group what pieces of the First Place 4 Health program still baffle them. Record their answers on a whiteboard or flip chart.

Have one or two members of your group talk about how Abraham's journey of faith parallels their First Place 4 Health journey. Be sure they include both victories and struggles—and mistakes—in their story. You might want to ask the members before the meeting so that they can think about the parallels before they speak to the group.

Abraham and Sarah laughed to themselves when God spoke about their son to come, not because they were overjoyed, but because they thought God was joking! Ask your group to identify times they have laughed at God's Word because it seemed impossible.

Talk about how "Is anything too hard for the Lord?" can be part of our First Place 4 Health journey.

During our Day Six reflection time, we looked at names society gives people carrying excess body weight. On your flip chart or whiteboard, record the names your group came up with during the exercise. Then ask your group to talk about the new names God will give them as they step forward in faith.

Ask members to share their altars from the Day Seven project. Be sure each person has an opportunity to explain why they picked the 12 words or phrases they put inside the rocks.

## week four: receptive to the Word

As you begin today's session, please lead a discussion about the difference between "press on" and "press in" as it applies to First Place 4 Health.

On your whiteboard or flip chart, write down the feelings and emotions that your group has identified as being stirred when they hear the words "press in."

This week we studied the Parable of the Sower. Ask one person in your group to read aloud Mark 4:4-8 and another to read aloud Mark 4:15-20. Then lead a discussion on how the "birds" gobble up the Word seed in those areas of our heart that are packed down by the things of this world. Go on a "bird hunt" and identify those things that can snatch away the Word seed before it can germinate and take root.

Starting a diet and exercise program is easy. Perseverance is the challenge. Ask your group how starting strong and falling away is like the second type of seed. Record their answers on a whiteboard or flip chart.

It is important that your group members are able to recognize the three things that choke out the Word and make it unfruitful to their First Place 4 Health program. Talk about each of the things that our memory verse tells us can sabotage our progress.

Be sure to include time to talk about the solution rather than focus on the problem! Ask your group what ways they identified to press on.

Day Five provides an excellent opportunity to talk about the different results each First Place 4 Health member will have. Talk about the importance of each person doing his or her best—and then leaving the results to God.

On Day Seven your group went on a nature hike. Allow each person an opportunity to show the items they collected and then talk about how each item spoke to them about a spiritual truth they've learned in their First Place 4 Health journey.

## week five: over it all

Have fun with the "layered-look" discussion that is in the introduction section of this week's study!

Talk about the importance of understanding what "all these virtues" spoken about in our memory verses consist of. Then list the seven virtues on a whiteboard or flip chart.

Our Day Two study asks us to apply these seven virtues to self-care. Lead a discussion on the ways your group discovered they could apply the seven virtues in Colossians 3:12-13 to self-care.

In order to put on these virtues, we must first eliminate our vices. Talk about the "old practices" that must be set aside before we can become a new creation in First Place 4 Health.

Psalm 32 gives us some graphic descriptions of what unconfessed sin can do to us physically, mentally, emotionally and spiritually. Talk about how David describes the consequences of not confessing one's sins.

Fortunately, confession changes all that is described in Psalm 32. Ahead of time, ask a member of your group—someone who is willing to be transparent and vulnerable—to talk to the group about a time confession of a sin brought relief. (That someone can be you!)

On Day Six we looked at binge foods. Give each person in your group an opportunity to share at least one binge food and the healthy, life-giving food they will replace it with.

Using the Day Seven exercise as your example, talk about how we can be at war with ourselves over participation in First Place 4 Health. But don't spend all your time discussing the problem. Talk about how we can solve the "at war with self" dilemma.

## week six: pursuit presses on

Our memory verse for Week Six, like the Week Five verse, needs to be put in the context in which it was written in order to understand what is being said. Talk to your group about the importance of always keeping a verse anchored to the text in which it appears.

This week we learned about the "rule of five" as it applies to Bible interpretation. List the five elements of the "rule of five" and post them in the room during this study.

Our memory verse comes from 1 Timothy 6 and our study looked at verses 3 through 10. Ask your group to identify the problem Paul was addressing in this passage and how that truth might apply to diets we tried before coming to First Place 4 Health.

Another valuable spiritual tool is called the principle of replacement. Lead a discussion about how our Week Five and Week Six memory verses have stressed the principle of replacement.

Talk about the impossibility of being a "secret service" Christian rather than a man or woman of God!

Use this discussion as a time to invite anyone in your group who has not already done so to make a *public* profession of faith.

Scripture contains many elements of paradox, and one of those is fleeing so that we can fight. Talk about why we must first flee before we can stand firm and fight.

Talk about the five elements of the "rule of five" and how your group has found each element to be helpful in their understanding of this week's memory verse.

Tell the group to continue to use the "rule of five" in their personal Bible reading and Scripture memory practices.

Have group members share the five ways they will apply this week's memory verse to their First Place 4 Health efforts. Record their answers on a whiteboard or flip chart.

End today's session with a time of "selah"—taking five minutes to meditate on God's goodness and grace in Christ Jesus our Lord.

## week seven: all who run can win

We have passed the halfway mark in the *Moving Forward Together* Bible study. Begin this session with a time of review, asking your group to recap what they learned in each of the first five weeks of the study.

Talk to the group about the "all who run can win" concept and how each of us only competes against our prior level of achievement as we strive to do our personal best.

Paul was compelled to preach the gospel, and so are we! As part of your Day Two study, your group was asked to reach out to one person in need of First Place 4 Health. Have your group report on their efforts—and the result of those efforts.

We are training in all four facets of our being in First Place 4 Health. Lead a discussion on what type of training we are doing in each aspect of our being. You might want to list the four aspects (physical, mental, emotional and spiritual) on your whiteboard or flip chart as you lead this discussion.

We are to store up treasures in heaven. How is storing up treasures in heaven part of the motivation to achieve First Place 4 Health success? Ask your group this question and record on your whiteboard or flip chart the answers you get.

Spend plenty of time talking about the Day Five study. All too often people use verses like 1 Corinthians 9:27 as an excuse to mistreat the body God created and calls good.

Our Day Six reflection contained the story of a high-jump competitor. Lead a discussion with your group about throwing their "heart over the bar" and what that looks like in First Place 4 Health.

Ask members of your group to share their experience as they did the Day Seven exercise. End your session by going around the room and having each person say this week's memory verse out loud, each one placing emphasis on the next word in the verse, like we did in Day Seven.

## week eight: true glory

Maturity is an asset in the kingdom of God. Spend some time talking to your group about the benefits of spiritual maturity.

Our memory verse for this week was written to elders in the Church. Are you, as the group leader, a living example of the First Place 4 Health program? Talk to your group about this!

How was Jesus, the Good Shepherd, different from the false teachers who led their flock astray? Put "Good Shepherd" and "False Teachers" on your whiteboard or flip chart, and have the group tell you how they are different.

Jeremiah 9:23-24 contains some wonderful words about what the real source of our glory needs to be. Lead a group discussion about the three things, according to Jeremiah, that are not to be a source of boasting and pride. Write the three things on your whiteboard or flip chart. Talk about how each of these is a detriment to progress in First Place 4 Health.

Humbling ourselves under God's mighty hand brings up unpleasant memories for those who have suffered abuse at the cruel hands of authority figures. Talk about how the Good Shepherd tenderly cares for His flock.

Although we have been looking at analogies about athletes, particularly athletic prizes and crowns, Jesus gives us another perspective of our reward in heaven in the Parable of the Talents. Talk about what it is like to enter into the Master's happiness and how that is different from a tangible reward.

There will undoubtedly be folks in your group who still think they can work or run hard enough to earn salvation. Spend lots of time on the Ephesians 2:4-10 questions of Day Five.

Ask one or two of the members of your group, those who will be honest and transparent, to share what their accounting before God would look like if the

Master returned tonight. Please ask them to make their accounting specific to First Place 4 Health.

Review with your group the questions from the Day Seven reflection. Ask someone to record the group's answers on a whiteboard or flip chart.

# week nine: breaking free

Using the story about having the wrong roadmap (given in the introduction to this week's study), talk about how we cannot get to our desired goal without a proper interpretation of Scripture.

Hebrews 11:6 tells us that God rewards those who earnestly seek Him. Lead a discussion about what earnestly seeking God through the First Place 4 Health program means and what the reward is that we are promised.

Ask your group if they *really* believe Hebrews 11:6 at a heart level, and if not, why not.

Hindrances are external things that keep us from running the race marked out for us. On your whiteboard or flip chart, write down the things your group identified as hindrances. Now ask them how they plan to throw off those hindrances, and record those answers, too.

Sins are not only substantial acts but also insubstantial inner attitudes and beliefs that leave us vulnerable. Talk about the insubstantial "sins" that comprise "the sin that so easily entangles" us.

Members were asked to encourage someone in the group as part of the Day Three lesson. Ask those who received encouragement to talk about how good it felt to receive heartening words that bolstered their confidence.

Put the words "speed" and "perseverance" on your whiteboard or flip chart, and talk about the difference between these two things.

It is important for your group to realize that although we all have the same goal (Christian maturity, which includes health and wholeness), we each run a different course to reach that goal. Use the variety of Olympic events as a means to talk about how each person has different gifts and talents and so must "run their race" different from how others strive to reach their goal.

Day Six talks about balance. Ask two or three members of your group to share about how God has worked in their life physically, mentally, emotionally and spiritually during this session of First Place 4 Health. In that discussion, ask them to include how God worked in the weakest area in order to help bring balance and harmony.

Ask the group members to identify one behavior or belief they have eliminated during this session of First Place 4 Health—and what they replaced it with.

## week ten: focused on the prize

Have someone in your group read Luke 4:18-19 to the group. Then ask each group member to identify the healing ministry of Jesus they need most in their life right now—and tell why they selected that one.

The memory verses for Weeks Nine and Ten have three "Let Us" statements in them. List all three on the whiteboard or flip chart, and talk about how each one of them is part of First Place 4 Health.

When Jesus encountered the blind man on the road, His disciples wanted to blame the man or his parents for the malady. Ask your group to talk about blaming others for the problems that brought them to First Place 4 Health.

Lead a discussion about how our out-of-control eating can be used to manifest God's glory when we are healed and restored.

Have a group member read aloud the account of the snake on the pole (Numbers 21:4-9). Then talk to your group about what caused God to send the snakes—and what "snakes" are ours when we grumble and complain against God.

Ask someone to read aloud the story of the bent woman (Luke 13:10-17) and another to read aloud the story of the demon-possessed boy (Mark 9:17-27). Then, talk to your group about the difference between being crippled by a spirit and being possessed by a demon!

Ask each person to identify one area of their life that is crippled by a spirit and in need of Jesus' healing touch.

Concern for loved ones is a major distraction to our First Place 4 Health efforts. Rather than emphasizing the extent of the infirmity of the demon-possessed boy, emphasize how the father kept his eyes focused on Jesus—the solution, not the problem!

End your meeting with a time of prayer for loved ones who are out of control. Then pray for the members of your group who need to look to Jesus rather than be consumed by the problems of their loved ones.

## week eleven: binding it all together

On a whiteboard or flip chart divided into two columns, write "The Root of Bitterness" over one column. Ask the members of your group to name some of the ways bitterness has stood in the way of their physical, emotional, mental and spiritual health.

Read aloud Exodus 15:22-25, or ask a volunteer to read it. Remind the group that the piece of wood Moses threw into the water can symbolize the cross. Write "The Cross of Christ" over the second column. Ask your members to share how the cross has turned their bitterness into sweetness and list their answers in the column.

Ask a volunteer to read Romans 12:17-19 aloud. Ask members to share how their concept of the importance of forgiveness has changed through the past week's Bible study.

Break the group into pairs. Ask the members to share with their partner about a time, past or present, when they have had difficulty forgiving someone. Have each partner pray for the other. Plan 7 to 10 minutes for this exercise.

When the group comes together again, talk about our appropriate response to God's grace demonstrated through Christ's death, as explored in Day Three. Ask the group to sit in silence for 1 or 2 minutes as they consider whether or not they are responding wholeheartedly. End the time of silence in prayer, thanking God for putting our sin to death on the cross, and asking for His strength to press on.

At the end of your prayer, instead of saying "Amen," say Philippians 4:4: "Rejoice in the Lord always. I will say it again: Rejoice!" Invite the group to say it with you several times, and raise the volume until everyone is shouting and rejoicing! Challenge your group to forgive and rejoice throughout the coming week.

## week twelve: time to celebrate!

Even though most of your meeting this week will be a victory celebration, take time to talk about how much God loves us and how we are called to love our brothers and sisters in Christ because God loves us. (See "Planning a Victory Celebration" in the *First Place 4 Health Leader's Guide* for ideas about throwing a successful celebration for your group.)

Spend the rest of the study time allowing each member to tell their *Moving Forward Together* story. Give members an equal opportunity to share the good things God has done for them in this First Place 4 Health session. Don't allow the more talkative group members to monopolize all the time. Even the quiet members need an opportunity to share their stories! Even those who have not lost weight (and there may even be a few who have gained weight) have still been part of the journey, so allow them to share their story and talk about why they did not succeed.

Making a commitment to continue in First Place 4 Health is an important part of victory. Be sure to talk about your group's future plans, and make each person feel welcome to continue to journey with you.

End your victory celebration by reading aloud Hebrews 13:20-21, a wonderful benediction.

# First Place 4 Health
# menu plans

Each menu plan is based on approximately 1,400 to 1,500 calories per day. All recipe and menu exchanges were determined using the MasterCook software, a program that accesses a database containing more than 6,000 food items prepared using the United States Department of Agriculture (USDA) publications and information from food manufacturers. As with any nutritional program, MasterCook calculates the nutritional values of the recipes based on ingredients. Nutrition may vary due to how the food is prepared, where the food comes from, soil content, season, ripeness, processing and method of preparation. For these reasons, please use the recipes and menu plans as approximate guides. As always, consult your physician and/or a registered dietitian before starting a weight-loss program.

*For those who need more calories, add the following to the 1,400-calorie plan:*

- 1,800 calories: 2 ounce equivalent of meat, 3 ounce equivalent of bread, $1/2$ cup vegetable serving, 1 tsp. fat

- 2,000 calories: 2 ounce equivalent of meat, 4 ounce equivalent of bread, $1/2$ cup vegetable serving, 3 tsp. fat

- 2,200 calories: 2 ounce equivalent of meat, 5 ounce equivalent of bread, $1/2$ cup vegetable serving, $1/2$ cup fruit serving, 5 tsp. fat

- 2,400 calories: 2 ounce equivalent of meat, 6 ounce equivalent of bread, 1 cup vegetable serving, $1/2$ cup fruit serving, 6 tsp. fat

# First Week Grocery List

## Produce
- ❐ (1) white onion
- ❐ (1) bell pepper
- ❐ (5) oranges
- ❐ (1) cantaloupe
- ❐ (2) peaches
- ❐ (2) bananas
- ❐ potatoes
- ❐ green beans
- ❐ (3) apples
- ❐ (30) spears fresh asparagus
- ❐ 4 cups broccoli
- ❐ 4 cups berries
- ❐ large bag spinach leaves
- ❐ (1) bag baby carrots
- ❐ (1) bunch celery stalks
- ❐ (2) small plums
- ❐ (1) bunch green leaf lettuce
- ❐ (1) package fresh mushrooms
- ❐ 2 cups strawberries
- ❐ 2 cups mixed greens
- ❐ (3) red peppers
- ❐ (1) package grapes
- ❐ (1) red onion
- ❐ (6) roma tomatoes
- ❐ (1) bunch romaine lettuce leaves

## Baking Products
- ❐ cinnamon
- ❐ nutmeg
- ❐ walnuts
- ❐ (1) jar applesauce
- ❐ Tabasco sauce
- ❐ garlic salt
- ❐ nonstick cooking spray
- ❐ reduced-fat Miracle Whip®

- ❐ reduced-fat Ranch dressing
- ❐ ground pepper
- ❐ dried oregano
- ❐ ground nutmeg
- ❐ balsamic vinegar
- ❐ salt
- ❐ olive oil
- ❐ Italian bread crumbs
- ❐ flour
- ❐ raisins
- ❐ (1) jar salsa
- ❐ all-fruit strawberry spread
- ❐ fresh lemon or lime juice
- ❐ pasta
- ❐ grape juice
- ❐ brown rice
- ❐ reduced-fat Catalina-style dressing
- ❐ 6 oz. wide egg noodles (whole-wheat blend)
- ❐ light Italian dressing
- ❐ red wine vinegar

## Breads and Cereals
- ❐ nonfat whole-wheat flour tortillas
- ❐ whole-wheat pita bread
- ❐ Grape Nuts
- ❐ Rice Chex®
- ❐ English muffins
- ❐ instant oatmeal (flavored, sugar-free)
- ❐ saltine crackers
- ❐ French bread
- ❐ breadsticks
- ❐ oyster crackers
- ❐ low-calorie rye bread
- ❐ Italian bread
- ❐ oatmeal

## Canned Foods

- ❐ (1) 15 $\frac{1}{2}$-oz. can red salmon
- ❐ (1) 2-oz. jar pimientos
- ❐ (1) jar marinara sauce
- ❐ (1) can white beans
- ❐ (1) can condensed beef broth
- ❐ (1) can vegetable soup
- ❐ (1) can wax beans
- ❐ (1) can chickpeas
- ❐ (2) cans sliced peaches in fruit juice
- ❐ (1) small can black olives
- ❐ (1) 10 $\frac{3}{4}$-oz. can reduced-fat Cream of Mushroom soup

## Dairy Products

- ❐ light margarine
- ❐ nonfat milk
- ❐ egg substitute
- ❐ (1) sugar-free nonfat yogurt with fruit
- ❐ $\frac{1}{4}$ cup 2%-fat cottage cheese
- ❐ light mayonnaise
- ❐ 4 oz. light sour cream

- ❐ 2 oz. reduced-fat cheddar cheese
- ❐ eggs
- ❐ 2-oz. part-skim mozzarella cheese
- ❐ reduced-fat feta cheese

## Seafood and Meat

- ❐ (1) 10-oz. Lean Cuisine Dinner Selects
- ❐ (4) 4-oz. pork center loin
- ❐ 1 lb. red snapper
- ❐ 12 $\frac{1}{2}$ oz. boneless skinless chicken breasts
- ❐ 1 lb. extra-lean ground beef
- ❐ (2) 8-oz. lean strip loin steaks (1″ thick)

## Frozen Foods

- ❐ whole-wheat waffles
- ❐ (1) 16-oz. bag frozen dark-pitted cherries
- ❐ (2) 10-oz. pkg. frozen asparagus
- ❐ sugar-free, nonfat chocolate yogurt

# First Week Meals and Recipes

## DAY 1

### Breakfast

2 whole-grain waffles
1 cup nonfat milk

2 tbsp. raisins
$1/2$ cup applesauce, sweetened with
    artificial sweetener (if desired)

*Nutritional Information:* 397 calories (16% calories from fat); 6g fat; 19g protein; 52g carbohydrate; 6g dietary fiber; 4mg cholesterol; 132mg sodium.

### Lunch

#### Broiled Chicken Breasts

$2^1/2$-oz. boneless, skinless
    chicken breast, broiled and
    served with mixed bean salad
$1/2$ cup Italian green beans, cooked

$1/2$ cup chickpeas, drained
$1/2$ cup wax beans
1 tbsp. reduced-fat Italian dressing

Serve each with 2 breadsticks, $1/2$ teaspoon margarine and 1 small nectarine.

*Nutritional Information:* 509 calories (14% calories from fat); 10g fat; 34g protein; 103g carbohydrate; 12g dietary fiber; 41mg cholesterol; 1,595mg sodium.

### Dinner

#### Italian Breaded Snapper

1 lb. red snapper, cut into 4 fillets
$1/2$ tsp. salt
1 tbsp. olive oil

1 tbsp. fresh lemon or lime juice
$1/2$ cup Italian-seasoned breadcrumbs

Rinse fish fillets and pat dry with paper towel. Combine breadcrumbs with salt in small plate. Dip fillets in lemon or lime juice, and then dip in breadcrumbs to coat. Heat oil in large nonstick skillet. Cook fillets over medium heat 4 to 5 minutes each side, turning once (about 10 minutes total for 1-inch thick fillets or until flakey when tested with fork). Serve each with 1 cup steamed broccoli, $1/2$ cup cooked pasta tossed with $1/4$ cup prepared marinara sauce, 1 breadstick and 1 cup mixed berries. Serves 4.

*Nutritional information:* 497 calories (15% calories from fat); 9g fat; 39g protein; 79g carbohydrate; 11g dietary fiber; 42mg cholesterol; 1,407mg sodium.

# DAY 2

### Breakfast

1 package flavored instant oatmeal (no sugar added)
2 walnut halves, chopped
1 small banana
1 cup nonfat milk

*Nutritional Information:* 519 calories (13% calories from fat); 8g fat; 23g protein; 92g carbohydrate; 12g dietary fiber; 4mg cholesterol; 945mg sodium.

### Lunch

#### Mozzarella Sandwich

2 oz. reduced-fat mozzarella cheese
$1/4$ cup roasted red bell pepper,
   cut into strips
1 tsp. red wine vinegar
2 1-oz. slices Italian bread, toasted
$1/4$ cup romaine lettuce leaves
2 slices tomato
$1^1/2$ tsp. light Italian dressing
1 cup whole green beans, cooked and
   chilled

Drizzle vinegar and dressing over bell peppers and tomato slices. Layer cheese, lettuce, bell pepper and tomato between bread slices. Serve with chilled green beans and 1 small orange.

*Nutritional Information:* 407 calories (28% calories from fat); 13g fat; 24g protein; 53g carbohydrate; 9g dietary fiber; 31mg cholesterol; 619mg sodium.

### Dinner

#### Ground Beef Stroganoff on Noodles

6 oz. egg-free noodles
1 lb. extra-lean ground beef
1 medium onion, diced
1 tsp. flour
$1/2$ tsp. ground pepper
1 cup beef broth
1 tbsp. reduced-fat margarine
8 oz. mushrooms, sliced
$1/2$ tsp. salt
$1/4$ cup reduced-fat sour cream

Cook noodles according to package directions (omitting salt and fat); then drain and combine with $1/2$ cup beef broth in medium cooking pot. Cook ground beef in skillet over medium heat until well done. Drain and remove from skillet; set aside. Sauté onions and mushrooms in margarine for 3 minutes, or until tender crisp. Sprinkle with flour and season with salt and pepper. Add remaining beef broth and bring mixture to a boil. Simmer for 2 minutes. Add cooked ground beef and slowly stir in sour cream. Return to heat and cook over low heat until warm—*do not* let boil or sour cream will curdle. Serve over noodles. Serve each with a spinach salad with $^1/_4$ cup sliced strawberries and 1 tablespoon reduced-fat sweet and sour dressing. Serves 4.

*Nutritional Information:* 494 calories (42% calories from fat); 23g fat; 32g protein; 39g carbohydrate; 3g dietary fiber; 120mg cholesterol; 723mg sodium.

## DAY 3

### Breakfast

$^3/_4$ cup Rice Chex (or other unsweetened fortified dried cereal)
$^1/_2$ English muffin
1 tsp. all-fruit spread
1 small banana
$^1/_2$ tsp. reduced-fat margarine
1 cup nonfat milk

*Nutritional Information:* 381 calories (6% calories from fat); 3g fat; 13g protein; 78g carbohydrate; 4g dietary fiber; 4mg cholesterol; 491mg sodium.

### Lunch

*Egg Salad Sandwich*
1 egg, hard-boiled and minced
$^1/_4$ cup celery, chopped
2 slices reduced-calorie rye bread
1 egg white, hard-boiled and minced
2 tsp. reduced-calorie mayonnaise

Combine minced eggs, celery and mayonnaise. Spread on bread to make sandwich. Serve with 1 cup each carrot sticks and zucchini, 2 tablespoons reduced-fat Ranch dressing and 4 ounces sugar-free, nonfat, chocolate-flavored frozen yogurt.

*Nutritional Information:* 388 calories (23% calories from fat); 10g fat; 20g protein; 60g carbohydrate; 15g dietary fiber; 221mg cholesterol; 547mg sodium.

### Dinner

*Pizza Hut Supreme Pizza*
2 slices medium Thin and Crispy Supreme
Tossed with salad with 1 tbsp. salad dressing

Serve with 1 cup sliced peaches, drained.

*Nutritional Information:* 548 calories (52% calories from fat); 44g fat; 24g protein; 65g carbohydrate; 7g dietary fiber; 60mg cholesterol; 1,470mg sodium.

# DAY 4

........................................................................................

## Breakfast

### *Breakfast Burrito*

(2) 6-inch fat-free flour tortillas
2 tbsp. onion, chopped
2 tbsp. salsa

$^1/_2$ cup egg substitute, scrambled
2 tbsp. bell pepper, chopped

Serve with 1 small orange

*Nutritional Information:* 455 calories (30% calories from fat); 16g fat; 22g protein; 60g carbo-hydrate; 6g dietary fiber; 2mg cholesterol; 941mg sodium.

........................................................................................

## Lunch

### *Soup and Salad*

(1) 8-oz. can vegetable soup (90-calorie), served with
2 cups mixed green lettuce
$^1/_2$ cup celery, sliced
2 oz. reduced-fat cheddar cheese, diced

$^1/_2$ cup roasted red bell pepper strips, chilled
1 tbsp. light Italian dressing
1 tsp. light margarine
(1) 1-oz. slice Italian or French bread

Serve with 20 oyster crackers and 1 cup strawberries.

*Nutritional Information:* 449 calories (23% calories from fat); 12g fat; 25g protein; 64g carbo-hydrate; 12g dietary fiber; 12mg cholesterol; 1,549mg sodium.

........................................................................................

## Dinner

### *Pork Chops with Cherry Sauce*

(4) 4-oz. boneless, center-cut pork chops, trimmed of fat
$^1/_2$ tsp. garlic salt
$^3/_4$ tsp. dried leaf oregano, crushed
$^1/_2$ tsp. ground nutmeg
$^1/_2$ tsp. balsamic vinegar

nonstick cooking spray
$^1/_2$ tsp. ground pepper
(1) 16-oz. bag frozen dark-red pitted cherries, thawed and drained
$^1/_2$ cup red grape juice

Coat a large skillet with nonstick cooking spray. Coat pork chops evenly on both sides with garlic salt and pepper. Arrange in preheated skillet and brown well on both sides over medium heat. Combine grape juice, vinegar, remaining seasonings and half of cherries in blender. Puree and pour over pork chops in skillet. Sprinkle remaining cherries over top, and then reduce heat. Cover and simmer 10 minutes. Serve each immediately with $^1/_3$ cup cooked brown rice, 6 to 8 steamed asparagus spears and a slice of garlic bread with $^1/_2$ teaspoon reduced-fat margarine. Serves 4.

*Nutritional Information:* 429 calories (27% calories from fat); 13g fat; 25g protein; 54g carbohydrate; 5g dietary fiber; 56mg cholesterol; 665mg sodium.

# DAY 5

## Breakfast

1 cup oatmeal with
1/4 tsp. reduced-fat margarine
dash nutmeg
1 cup nonfat milk

dash cinnamon
2 tbsp. raisins

*Nutritional Information:* 284 calories (11% calories from fat); 3g fat; 15g protein; 50g carbohydrate; 5g dietary fiber; 4mg cholesterol; 517mg sodium.

## Lunch

### Burger King Kid's Meal
1 small hamburger (without mayonnaise)
1 small French Fries
1 small diet soda

Serve with 1 small apple.

*Nutritional Information:* 575 calories (38% calories from fat); 25g fat; 17g protein; 77g carbohydrate; 7g dietary fiber; 40mg cholesterol; 945mg sodium.

## Dinner

### Salmon Cakes
(1) 15 1/2-oz. can red salmon, drained
(1) 2-oz. jar diced pimentos
3 tbsp. reduced-fat Miracle Whip
3 drops Tabasco sauce
2 tsp. onion, minced

6 saltines, crushed
1 tsp. lemon juice
Butter-flavored nonstick cooking spray

Remove skin and large bones from fish. Combine remaining ingredients in medium mixing bowl, mashing any remaining bones with a fork. Shape mixture into 4 patties. Coat medium skillet with nonstick cooking spray. Cook salmon cakes over medium-high heat until lightly browned on each side. Serve with 1/2 cup garlic mashed potatoes, 1 cup green beans and a medium piece of fruit. Serves 4.

*Nutritional Information:* 496 calories (28% calories from fat); 18g fat; 50g protein; 54g carbohydrate; 10g dietary fiber; 124mg cholesterol; 624mg sodium.

# DAY 6

## Breakfast

### Breakfast Pita

(1) 6-inch whole-wheat pocket pita
$1/3$ cup diced peaches, in own juice

$1/4$ cup 2% cottage cheese
2 walnuts, chopped

Combine cottage cheese, peaches and walnuts. Split pita in half; fill each half with cottage cheese mixture.

*Nutritional Information:* 290 calories (22% calories from fat); 8g fat; 20g protein; 44g carbohydrate; 8g dietary fiber; 5mg cholesterol; 570mg sodium.

## Lunch

### Spinach, Bean and Chicken Salad

2 cups spinach leaves
$1/4$ cup cooked cannelloni
  (white kidney) beans, drained

2 oz. skinless, boneless chicken
  breast, cooked and diced
2 tbsp. reduced-fat Catalina-style dressing

Serve with $1/2$ cup each carrot and celery sticks, 2 long breadsticks and 2 small plums.

*Nutritional Information:* 322 calories (24% calories from fat); 9g fat; 27g protein; 35g carbohydrate; 9g dietary fiber; 39mg cholesterol; 318mg sodium.

## Dinner

### Grecian Skillet Steaks

(2) 8-oz. lean strip loin steaks,
  about 1-inch thick
$11/2$ tsp. dried leaf oregano, crushed
$1/2$ tsp. salt
1 tbsp. olive oil
2 tbsp. feta cheese, crumbled

1 tbsp. ripe olives, chopped
1 tsp. dried leaf basil, crushed
$1/4$ tsp. black pepper
3 garlic cloves, minced
1 tbsp. fresh lemon juice

Sprinkle both sides of steaks with herbs and seasonings. Heat oil on medium heat in large skillet. Add garlic and sauté for 1 minute. Add steaks and cook 5 minutes on each side for medium-rare (longer for well-done). Remove from heat and sprinkle with cheese, lemon juice and olives. Cut each steak in half before serving. Serve each with $1/2$ cup roasted potatoes, 1 cup marinated green beans, a 1-ounce dinner roll and 1 small orange. Serves 4.

*Nutritional Information:* 626 calories (45% calories from fat); 32g fat; 30g protein; 58g carbohydrate; 10g dietary fiber; 83mg cholesterol; 866mg sodium.

# DAY 7

## Breakfast

$1/3$ medium cantaloupe or honeydew
1 cup artificially sweetened, nonfat pineapple-flavored yogurt
$1/4$ cup Grape Nuts

*Nutritional Information:* 320 calories (4% calories from fat); 1g fat; 14g protein; 50g carbohydrate; 5g dietary fiber; 3mg cholesterol; 256mg sodium.

## Lunch

### Frozen Light Dinner Entree

(1) 10- to 11-ounce frozen light dinner entrée (with 300 to 350 calories, fewer than 800 mg sodium and fewer than 10 grams fat)

Spinach salad with mushrooms
1 tbsp. reduced-calorie dressing

Serve with 15 grapes.

*Nutritional Information:* 421 calories (10% calories from fat); 5g fat; 24g protein; 74g carbohydrate; 9g dietary fiber; 40mg cholesterol; 632mg sodium.

## Dinner

### Asparagus Chicken

$1/2$ lb. chicken tenders
(1) $10^3/4$-oz. can reduced-fat cream of mushroom soup
1 tsp. lemon juice
$3/4$ cup reduced-fat cheddar cheese, shredded

(2) 10-oz. pkg. frozen asparagus, thawed
$1/2$ cup reduced-fat mayonnaise
Dash cayenne pepper
$1/4$ cup seasoned breadcrumbs
Butter-flavored nonstick cooking spray

Preheat oven to 375° F. Coat 8x8-inch baking dish and large skillet each with nonstick cooking spray. Sauté $1/2$ chicken in skillet 1 to 2 minutes; remove and repeat with remaining chicken. Place asparagus in bottom of baking dish. Arrange chicken over asparagus. Combine soup, mayonnaise, lemon juice and pepper in medium bowl. Pour into skillet and heat until bubbly, stirring constantly. Pour over chicken. Top with cheese and bake for 15 minutes, covered. Remove cover and sprinkle with breadcrumbs, then bake 10 more minutes. Serve with $1/2$ cup cooked rice and 1 small apple. Serves 4.

*Nutritional Information:* 421 calories (10% calories from fat); 5g fat; 24g protein; 74g carbohydrate; 9g dietary fiber; 40mg cholesterol; 632mg sodium.

## Second Week Grocery List

### Produce

- ❑ (2) packages fresh mushrooms
- ❑ (2) onions
- ❑ (2) grapefruits
- ❑ (1) peach
- ❑ (1) package strawberries
- ❑ (2) plums
- ❑ (2) bunches broccoli
- ❑ garlic cloves
- ❑ (1) bunch scallions
- ❑ (1) bunch cauliflower
- ❑ (3) bananas
- ❑ (1) bag mixed greens
- ❑ (1) bag potatoes
- ❑ 5 cups fresh green beans
- ❑ cantaloupe or other type melon to make 3 cups
- ❑ (1) bunch fresh cilantro
- ❑ (3) cucumbers
- ❑ (1) green bell pepper
- ❑ (1) red bell pepper
- ❑ (2) kiwi fruits
- ❑ (1) head of cabbage
- ❑ (1) bag baby carrots
- ❑ (2) apples
- ❑ (4) tomatoes
- ❑ (1) head romaine lettuce
- ❑ (1) bunch celery
- ❑ (1) bunch grapes
- ❑ (1) cup berries
- ❑ (1) small bunch alfalfa sprouts
- ❑ (1) package raspberries

### Dairy Products

- ❑ eggs
- ❑ nonfat milk
- ❑ 2 oz. reduced-fat cheddar cheese
- ❑ (3) packages nonfat sugar-free yogurt with fruit
- ❑ 6 oz. nonfat plain yogurt
- ❑ (1) package light cream cheese
- ❑ Parmesan cheese
- ❑ light margarine
- ❑ 16-oz. package lowfat Swiss cheese
- ❑ 8 oz. part skim milk mozzarella cheese
- ❑ 6 oz. orange juice
- ❑ (1) small container lowfat, sugar-free vanilla yogurt

### Baking Products

- ❑ black pepper
- ❑ salt
- ❑ granulated garlic
- ❑ canned unsweetened applesauce
- ❑ raisins
- ❑ 6 oz. fettuccini noodles
- ❑ olive oil
- ❑ 16 oz. linguini noodles
- ❑ oregano
- ❑ ground nutmeg
- ❑ brown rice
- ❑ brown mustard
- ❑ honey
- ❑ $1/2$ cup pecans
- ❑ Italian seasoning
- ❑ all-purpose flour
- ❑ sugar
- ❑ rice
- ❑ 4 oz. wide noodles
- ❑ taco seasoning mix
- ❑ (1) jar chunky salsa

- ❏ nonstick cooking spray
- ❏ light Italian salad dressing
- ❏ pickle relish
- ❏ prepared mustard
- ❏ coleslaw dressing
- ❏ (1) package sugar-free orange gelatin
- ❏ light mayonnaise
- ❏ individual vanilla pudding
- ❏ (1) small jar roasted red peppers
- ❏ all-fruit strawberry spread

### Breads and Cereals
- ❏ (1) loaf whole-wheat bread
- ❏ small reduced-fat oat muffin
- ❏ box Grape Nuts
- ❏ box Kellogg's Nutri-Grain cereal
- ❏ bagels (2 oz. each)
- ❏ dinner rolls
- ❏ saltine crackers
- ❏ (1) package hot dog buns
- ❏ (1) small bag baked chips

### Meat and Seafood
- ❏ 1 lb. chicken tenders
- ❏ 3 lbs. boneless skinless chicken breasts
- ❏ 1 lb. tilapia
- ❏ 1 lb. round steaks

- ❏ (1) package reduced-fat hot dogs
- ❏ 2 oz. sliced roast beef
- ❏ (1) package turkey sausage

### Frozen Foods
- ❏ frozen waffles
- ❏ light pancakes
- ❏ (2) 10-oz. packages frozen chopped spinach
- ❏ (1) Lean Cuisine Dinner Selects
- ❏ (1) package frozen 100% fruit bars

### Canned Foods
- ❏ (1) 10-oz. can tomatoes with green chilies
- ❏ (1) can evaporated skim milk
- ❏ 32 oz. canned fruit salad in water
- ❏ (1) 10 $3/4$-oz. can reduced-fat condensed tomato soup
- ❏ (1) 15-oz. can chunky tomato sauce
- ❏ (1) 15-oz. can black beans
- ❏ (1) 8-oz. can beef barley soup
- ❏ (1) 4-oz. can pineapple in water
- ❏ (1) 14-oz. can peaches packed in juice
- ❏ (1) 8-oz. can tomato soup

## Second Week Meals and Recipes

# DAY 1

### Breakfast

1 slice whole-wheat (or 2 slices diet multigrain) bread, toasted
2 tsp. all-fruit spread
1 cup nonfat plain yogurt, artificially sweetened, garnished with
3 tbsp. wheat germ (or 2 tbsp. Grape Nuts)
6 oz. orange juice

*Nutritional Information:* 340 calories (5% calories from fat); 2g fat; 16g protein; 68g carbohydrate; 5g dietary fiber; 3mg cholesterol; 364mg sodium.

### Lunch

#### Roast Beef Sandwich

$1^1/_2$ oz. cooked lean, boneless roast beef, thinly sliced
1 tbsp. reduced-fat Thousand Island dressing

2 slices reduced-calorie bread
2 romaine lettuce leaves
2 slices tomato

Serve with $^1/_2$ cup each celery and carrot sticks, and 1 cup sugar-free white-grape flavored gelatin mixed with 1 cup grapes.

*Nutritional Information:* 416 calories (21% calories from fat); 9g fat; 25g protein; 50g carbohydrate; 7g dietary fiber; 36mg cholesterol; 1,018mg sodium.

### Dinner

#### Chicken Florentine

2 tsp. reduced-fat margarine
(1) $10^3/_4$-oz. can condensed reduced-fat cream of chicken soup, undiluted
2 oz. part-skim mozzarella cheese, shredded
(2) 10-oz. pkg. frozen chopped spinach

(4) 3-oz. boneless, skinless chicken breasts
$^1/_8$ tsp. ground nutmeg
$^1/_8$ tsp. ground black pepper
2 tbsp. fresh Parmesan cheese, grated

Preheat oven to 350° F. Melt margarine in large nonstick skillet over medium heat. Sauté chicken breasts 3 to 4 minutes on each side or until browned well. Combine soup, mozzarella and seasonings in medium saucepan. Cook over medium heat until cheese is melted. Line bottom of 13x9-inch baking dish with spinach. Top with chicken in a single layer. Pour cheese sauce evenly over the top; sprinkle with Parmesan cheese and bake for 12 to 15 minutes. Serve each with $1/3$ cup brown rice, 1 cup steamed cauliflower, a 1-ounce dinner roll and a banana. Serves 4.

*Nutritional Information:* 392 calories (35% calories from fat); 15g fat; 33g protein; 34g carbohydrate; 7g dietary fiber; 10mg cholesterol; 586mg sodium.

## DAY 2

### Breakfast

(1) 2-oz. whole-wheat bagel     1 tbsp. reduced-calorie cream cheese
3 medium stewed prunes (or 3 plums)     1 cup nonfat milk

*Nutritional Information:* 383 calories (12% calories from fat); 5g fat; 17g protein; 69g carbohydrate; 4g dietary fiber; 12mg cholesterol; 509mg sodium.

### Lunch

#### *Cheese and Veggie Sandwich with Tomato Soup*

(1) 8-oz. can ready-to-eat tomato soup     $1/4$ cup roasted red bell pepper strips,
$1/4$ cup alfalfa sprouts     drained
$1/4$ cup spinach leaves     1 oz. slice reduced-fat Swiss cheese
2 slices reduced-calorie whole-wheat     1 tbsp. reduced-fat Thousand Island
    bread     dressing

Serve with 6 saltine crackers, 1 cup broccoli florets and 1 cup artificially sweetened raspberry-flavored nonfat yogurt topped with $1/2$ cup raspberries.

*Nutritional Information:* 488 calories (18% calories from fat); 9g fat; 30g protein; 80g carbohydrate; 14g dietary fiber; 13mg cholesterol; 1,521mg sodium.

### Dinner

#### *Taco Beef and Pasta*

4 oz. rotini pasta, uncooked     1 lb. round-tip steak, about 1-inch thick
1 pkg. taco seasoning mix     1 tbsp. fresh cilantro, chopped
3 garlic cloves, crushed     1 tbsp. olive oil
2 cups chunky commercial salsa     (1) 15-oz. can black beans, rinsed and
$1/2$ cup water     drained

Cook pasta according to package directions (omitting fat). Cut steak into $1/4$-inch thick strips. Combine beef and seasonings; toss to coat. Heat skillet; then sauté half of steak strips over high heat 1 to 2 minutes, or until no longer pink. Remove from skillet with a slotted spoon; set aside. Sauté remaining half in same manner. Add pasta, salsa, beans and water to pan; cook 4 to 5 minutes over medium heat. Combine with beef in serving bowl and garnish as desired.

Serve each with salad of cucumbers and peppers, tossed with reduced-fat dressing, and 1 kiwi. Serves 4.

*Nutritional Information:* 541 calories (34% calories from fat); 20g fat; 34g protein; 54g carbohydrate; 10g dietary fiber; 67mg cholesterol; 1,590mg sodium.

## DAY 3

### Breakfast

(3) 4-inch lowfat pancakes
$1/2$ cup fresh strawberries, chopped

1 tsp. strawberry all-fruit spread
6 oz. nonfat plain yogurt

**Pancake topping:** Melt strawberry spread and combine with fresh strawberries and yogurt.

*Nutritional Information:* 262 calories (4% calories from fat); 1g fat; 14g protein; 49g carbohydrate; 2g dietary fiber; 3mg cholesterol; 305mg sodium.

### Lunch

*Arby's Turkey Deluxe Sandwich*
Green salad with fat-free dressing
Serve with $1/4$ cup canned peach slices, packed in own juice

*Nutritional Information:* 507 calories (31% calories from fat); 18g fat; 25g protein; 66g carbohydrate; 7g dietary fiber; 37mg cholesterol; 1,353mg sodium.

### Dinner

*Swiss-Style Chicken*

(3) 3-oz. boneless, skinless chicken breasts, cut into 16 strips
$3/4$ cup reduced-fat Swiss cheese, shredded
1 tsp. Italian seasoning
(1) 15-oz. can chunky tomato sauce
Butter-flavored nonstick cooking spray

2 tsp. reduced-fat margarine
1 garlic clove, minced
1 cup mushrooms, sliced
1 tbsp. all-purpose flour
2 tsp. sugar

Preheat oven to 350° F. Place chicken in 8x8-inch baking dish coated with nonstick cooking spray. Sprinkle chicken with cheese. Heat margarine in small skillet and sauté garlic 1 minute. Add mushrooms and sauté 2 to 3 minutes, or until tender. Combine tomato sauce, Italian seasoning, flour, sugar and mushrooms in small bowl; mix well and pour over cheese-topped chicken. Bake uncovered for 30 to 35 minutes. Serve with $1/4$ cup cooked rice and 1 cup broccoli. Serves 4.

*Nutritional Information:* 389 calories (28% calories from fat); 12g fat; 28g protein; 43g carbohydrate; 4g dietary fiber; 11mg cholesterol; 174mg sodium.

## DAY 4

### Breakfast

1 small reduced-fat oat muffin
1 medium fresh peach, or other fruit
1 cup artificially sweetened, nonfat fruit-flavored yogurt

*Nutritional Information:* 353 calories (14% calories from fat); 5g fat; 15g protein; 61g carbohydrate; 6g dietary fiber; 3mg cholesterol; 390mg sodium.

### Lunch

(1) 8-oz. can beef barley soup
6 saltine crackers
Dark green salad with vegetables and
3 tsp. reduced-fat dressing

Serve with 2 slices pineapple, packed in own juice.

*Nutritional Information:* 338 calories (31% calories from fat); 13g fat; 12g protein; 56g carbohydrate; 9g dietary fiber; 5mg cholesterol; 1,951mg sodium.

### Dinner

#### *Chicken Linguine*

12 oz. cooked boneless chicken breasts, cut into bite-sized pieces
4 oz. dry linguini
$1/2$ cup red bell peppers, chopped
1 cup mushrooms, sliced
2 garlic cloves, minced
1 tsp. dry leaf oregano, crushed
$1/2$ cup evaporated nonfat milk
$1/4$ cup fresh Parmesan cheese, shredded
1 tbsp. reduced-fat margarine
$1/2$ cup onion, chopped
4 oz. reduced-fat Jarlsberg or Swiss cheese, shredded
2 cups broccoli florets
$1/2$ cup scallions, sliced

Cook pasta according to package directions (omitting salt and fat). Drain and set aside. Melt margarine in large nonstick skillet and sauté peppers, onion, garlic, mushrooms and oregano. Cook for 5 minutes, stirring occasionally. Add chicken and remaining ingredients; then cook until cheese is melted, stirring constantly. Add linguini and mix well. Serves 4. (Refrigerate leftovers immediately for a great cold pasta salad.) Serve with 1 cup fruit salad mixed with 1 tablespoon lowfat vanilla yogurt.

*Nutritional Information:* 422 calories (20% calories from fat); 10g fat; 34g protein; 52g carbo-hydrate; 6g dietary fiber; 65mg cholesterol; 255mg sodium.

# DAY 5

......................................................................................................................

### Breakfast

*Brunch Casserole*

4 slices wheat bread, crusts removed
$1/4$ cup mushrooms, chopped
4 eggs, beaten (or 1 cup egg substitute)
$1/8$ tsp. black pepper
$1/8$ tsp. granulated garlic
Nonstick cooking spray

2 oz. turkey sausage
1 tsp. onion, chopped
1 cup nonfat milk
$1/4$ tsp. salt
2 oz. 2% cheddar cheese, shredded

Line bottom of 9x9-inch casserole dish with bread. Spray skillet with nonstick cooking spray. Sauté sausage until done. Remove from skillet and set aside. Sauté mushrooms and onions until tender. Crumble sausage and combine with mushrooms and onion. Sprinkle mixture over bread. Combine eggs, milk and seasonings and pour over top. Sprinkle with cheese. Cover and refrigerate overnight. Before cooking, set out for 15 minutes. Bake at 350° F for 40 to 45 minutes. Serve each with $1/2$ grapefruit. Serves 4.

*Nutritional Information:* 244 calories (32% calories from fat); 9g fat; 16g protein; 26g carbo-hydrate; 2g dietary fiber; 203mg cholesterol; 582mg sodium.

......................................................................................................................

### Lunch

2 oz. grilled fat-free hot dog
1 tsp. pickle relish
1 cup green and red cabbage, shredded
1 cup carrot sticks

(1) 2-oz. hot dog bread roll
1 tsp. prepared mustard
$1^1/2$ tsp. reduced-fat coleslaw dressing

Serve with 1 small apple.

*Nutritional Information:* 402 calories (15% calories from fat); 7g fat; 14g protein; 76g carbo-hydrate; 11g dietary fiber; 18mg cholesterol; 966mg sodium.

......................................................................................................................

### Dinner

*Spicy Chicken Stir-Fry Fettuccine*

6 oz. fettuccine noodles
3 garlic cloves, minced
1 lb. chicken tenders

2 tbsp. olive oil
$3/4$ tsp. black pepper
$1/2$ tsp. salt

8 oz. mushrooms, sliced

$^1/_4$ cup fresh Parmesan cheese, grated

(1) 10-oz. can diced tomatoes with green chiles

Cook pasta according to package directions (omitting salt and fat). Drain well and leave cooked pasta in pot. Mix oil, garlic and pepper in medium bowl; add chicken and toss to coat. Heat large nonstick skillet over medium heat and stir-fry chicken 2 to 3 minutes. Remove from skillet with slotted spoon and sprinkle with salt. Add mushrooms to skillet and stir-fry for 3 minutes. Add tomatoes and cooked chicken; stir well. Pour mixture into pot of pasta. Heat if needed. Add Parmesan and toss well. Serve each with 1 cup oven-roasted vegetables. Serves 4.

*Nutritional Information:* 395 calories (31% calories from fat); 9g fat; 9g protein; 38g carbohydrate; 3g dietary fiber; 80mg cholesterol; 367mg sodium.

# DAY 6

## Breakfast

1 cup Kellogg's Nutri-Grain cereal
1 cup nonfat milk
2 tbsp. raisins

*Nutritional Information:* 270 calories (2% calories from fat); 1g fat; 11g protein; 56g carbohydrate; 1g dietary fiber; 4mg cholesterol; 404mg sodium.

## Lunch

### Chicken Salad Sandwich

2 oz. cooked skinless, boneless chicken breast, chopped

$^1/_4$ cup celery, chopped

Pinch freshly ground black pepper

2 slices tomato

2 tsp. reduced-calorie mayonnaise

2 romaine lettuce leaves

2 slices reduced-calorie whole-wheat bread

Combine chicken, celery, mayonnaise and black pepper for sandwich filling. Spread on bread slices. Top with tomato and lettuce. Serve with $^1/_2$ cup each cucumber slices and carrot sticks, 1 small banana and $^1/_2$ cup reduced-calorie vanilla pudding (made with nonfat milk).

*Nutritional Information:* 384 calories (15% calories from fat); 7g fat; 9g protein; 79g carbohydrate; 9g dietary fiber; 12mg cholesterol; 528mg sodium.

## Dinner

### Honey-Mustard Pecan Tilapia

(4) 4-oz. tilapia, catfish or
   similar fish fillets
$1/4$ cup Creole or brown mustard
3 tsp. honey

2 tbsp. nonfat milk
1 cup pecans, or pecan meal, crushed
Nonstick cooking spray

Preheat oven to 450° F and coat sheet with nonstick cooking spray. Rinse fillets and pat dry. Combine mustard, milk and honey in small bowl. Dip fillets in milk mixture; then press into pecans to coat. Bake 12 minutes or until crisp. Serve each with $3/4$ cup mashed potatoes, 1 cup green beans and $3/4$ cup mixed melon balls. Serves 4.

*Nutritional Information:* 482 calories (41% calories from fat); 23g fat; 29g protein; 46g carbohydrate; 9g dietary fiber; 51mg cholesterol; 566mg sodium.

# DAY 7

## Breakfast

2 lowfat Eggo waffles
2 tbsp. raisins
1 cup nonfat milk

$1/2$ cup applesauce, sweetened with
   artificial sweetener (if desired)

*Nutritional Information:* 368 calories (15% calories from fat); 6g fat; 13g protein; 67g carbohydrate; 4g dietary fiber; 27mg cholesterol; 654mg sodium.

## Lunch

### Subway Veggie Delite

6-inch sandwich loaded with veggies with light mayonnaise

Serve with 1 cup mixed berries and 1 bag potato chips.

*Nutritional Information:* 404 calories (11% calories from fat); 6g fat; 14g protein; 100g carbohydrate; 12g dietary fiber; 0mg cholesterol; 801mg sodium.

## Dinner

### Frozen Dinner Entrée

(1) 10- to 11-oz. frozen dinner entrée
Tossed salad with veggies and 1 to 2 tbsp. reduced-fat dressing
1 frozen 100% juice bar

*Nutritional Information:* 359 calories (12% calories from fat); 5g fat; 23g protein; 57g carbohydrate; 10g dietary fiber; 40mg cholesterol; 608mg sodium.

## HEALTHY SNACK OPTIONS

- 2 skewers of *Fruit with Lemon-Lime Dip*: 160 calories (see recipe below)
- *Vegetable Salsa* with 14 pita chips: 150 calories (see recipe below)
- $1/2$ cup *Granola with Fruit and Cinnamon*: 163 calories (see recipe below)
- 30 small pretzel sticks: 90 calories
- 1 banana-chocolate whip (combine 1 cup fat-free milk, 1 small banana, a squeeze of chocolate syrup and a handful of ice cubes in a blender): 150 calories
- 3 cups air-popped popcorn sprinkled with 1 tablespoon Parmesan cheese: 120 calories
- 1 mini-bagel with fat-free cream cheese (2 oz.): 145 calories
- Snack Plate—25 red grapes, 3 tablespoons feta cheese, 6 crackers: 200 calories

(**Note**: You will need to add the ingredients for these items to the grocery lists.)


## SNACK RECIPES

### Fruit with Lemon-Lime Dip

4 ounces lowfat, sugar-free lemon yogurt 1 teaspoon fresh lime juice
1 teaspoon lime zest                     6 pineapple chunks
6 strawberries                           1 kiwi, peeled and diced
$1/2$ banana, cut into $1/2$-inch chunks   6 red grapes
4 wooden skewers

In a small bowl, whisk together the yogurt, lime juice and lime zest. Cover and refrigerate until needed. Thread 1 of each fruit onto the skewer. Repeat with the other skewers until the fruit is gone. Serve with the lemon-lime dip. Serves 2.

*Nutritional Information for two skewers:* 160 calories (6% calories from fat); 1g fat; 4g protein; 36g carbohydrate; 4g fiber; 4mg cholesterol; 45mg sodium; 122mg calcium.

### Vegetable Salsa

1 cup diced zucchini                       1 cup chopped red onion
2 red bell peppers, seeded and diced       2 green bell peppers, seeded and diced
4 tomatoes, diced                          2 garlic cloves, minced
$1/2$ cup chopped fresh cilantro             1 teaspoon ground black pepper
2 teaspoons sugar                          $1/4$ cup lime juice
1 teaspoon salt

Wash vegetables and prepare as directed. In a large bowl, combine all the ingredients. Toss gently to mix. Cover and refrigerate for at least 30 minutes to allow the flavors to blend. Serve with baked chips. (**Note:** For hotter salsa, add $1/2$ to 1 tablespoon finely chopped jalapeno peppers.)

*Nutritional Information for $^1/_2$ cup salsa:* 20 calories; 0g fat; 1g protein; 5g carbohydrate; 150mg sodium; 1g fiber; 12mg calcium.

### Granola with Fruit and Cinnamon

$^1/_4$ cup slivered almonds
$^1/_4$ cup unsweetened applesauce
1 tbsp. ground cinnamon
2 cups bran flakes
$^1/_2$ cup golden raisins

$^1/_4$ cup honey
1 tbsp. vanilla extract
2 cups dry old-fashioned oatmeal
$^3/_4$ cup dried apple pieces

Preheat oven to 325° F. Lightly coat a baking sheet with cooking spray. Spread the almonds on a baking sheet and bake, stirring occasionally, until golden and fragrant, about 10 minutes. Transfer immediately to a plate to cool. Raise the temperature of the oven to 350° F. In a small bowl, whisk together the honey, applesauce, vanilla and cinnamon. Set aside. In a large bowl, add the oatmeal and bran flakes. Stir to mix well. Add the honey mixture and toss with your hands. Don't break the clumps apart. Spread the cereal mixture evenly onto a baking sheet. Place in the oven and, stirring occasionally, bake until golden brown, about 30 minutes. Remove from the oven and cool slightly. In a large bowl, combine the cereal mixture, toasted almonds, apple pieces and raisins. Cool completely. Store in an airtight container.

*Nutritional Information per $^1/_2$ cup serving:* 163 calories (11% calories from fat); 2g fat; 4g protein; 33g carbohydrate; 4g fiber; 0mg cholesterol; 115mg sodium; 27mg calcium.

# Member Survey

Please answer the following questions to help your leader plan your First Place 4 Health meetings so that your needs might be met in this session. Give this form to your leader at the first group meeting.

Name _____    Birth date _____

Please list those who live in your household.

| Name | Relationship | Age |
|------|--------------|-----|
| _____ | _____ | _____ |
| _____ | _____ | _____ |
| _____ | _____ | _____ |
| _____ | _____ | _____ |

What church do you attend? _____

Are you interested in receiving more information about our church?

❏ Yes        ❏ No

Occupation _____

What talent or area of expertise would you be willing to share with our class?

_____

Why did you join First Place 4 Health?

_____

With notice, would you be willing to lead a Bible study discussion one week?

❏ Yes        ❏ No

Are you comfortable praying out loud? _____

If the assistant leader were absent, would you be willing to assist in weighing in members and possibly evaluating the Live It Trackers?

❏ Yes        ❏ No

Any other comments:

_____

_____

# Personal Weight and Measurement Record

| Week | Weight | + or - | Goal this Session | Pounds to goal |
|------|--------|--------|-------------------|----------------|
| 1 | | | | |
| 2 | | | | |
| 3 | | | | |
| 4 | | | | |
| 5 | | | | |
| 6 | | | | |
| 7 | | | | |
| 8 | | | | |
| 9 | | | | |
| 10 | | | | |
| 11 | | | | |
| 12 | | | | |

## Beginning Measurements

Waist _____ Hips _____ Thighs _____ Chest _____

## Ending Measurements

Waist _____ Hips _____ Thighs _____ Chest _____

# First Place 4 Health
## Prayer Partner

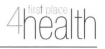

MOVING FORWARD
TOGETHER
Week
1

*I press on toward the goal to win the prize*
*for which God has called me heavenward in Christ Jesus.*

PHILIPPIANS 3:14

Date: _____

Name: _____

Home Phone: (_____) _____

Work Phone: (_____) _____

Email: _____

## Personal Prayer Concerns:

_____

_____

_____

_____

_____

_____

_____

This form is for prayer requests that are personal to you and your journey in First Place 4 Health. Please complete this form and have it ready to turn in when you arrive in class.

*First Place 4 Health*
*Prayer Partner*

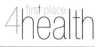

MOVING FORWARD
TOGETHER
Week
2

SCRIPTURE VERSE TO MEMORIZE FOR WEEK THREE:

*By faith Abraham, when called to go to a place he would later receive as his inheritance, obeyed and went, even though he did not know where he was going.*

HEBREWS 11:8

Date: _____

Name: _____

Home Phone: (_____) _____

Work Phone: (_____) _____

Email: _____

**Personal Prayer Concerns:**

_____

_____

_____

_____

_____

_____

_____

This form is for prayer requests that are personal to you and your journey in First Place 4 Health. Please complete this form and have it ready to turn in when you arrive at your group meeting.

# First Place 4 Health
## Prayer Partner

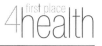

**MOVING FORWARD**
**TOGETHER**
Week
**3**

SCRIPTURE VERSE TO MEMORIZE FOR WEEK FOUR:

*But the worries of this life, the deceitfulness of wealth and the desires*
*for other things come in and choke the word, making it unfruitful.*

MARK 4:19

Date: _____

Name: _____

Home Phone: (_____)_____

Work Phone: (_____)_____

Email: _____

**Personal Prayer Concerns:**

_____

_____

_____

_____

_____

_____

_____

This form is for prayer requests that are personal to you and your journey in First Place 4 Health. Please complete this form and have it ready to turn in when you arrive at your group meeting.

# First Place 4 Health
## Prayer Partner

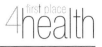

SCRIPTURE VERSE TO MEMORIZE FOR WEEK FIVE:

*And over all these virtues put on love,*
*which binds them all together in perfect unity.*

COLOSSIANS 3:14

Date: _____

Name: _____

Home Phone: (_____) _____

Work Phone: (_____) _____

Email: _____

**Personal Prayer Concerns:**

_____

_____

_____

_____

_____

_____

_____

This form is for prayer requests that are personal to you and your journey in First Place 4 Health. Please complete this form and have it ready to turn in when you arrive at your group meeting.

# First Place 4 Health
## Prayer Partner

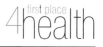

### MOVING FORWARD
### TOGETHER
#### Week
# 5

SCRIPTURE VERSE TO MEMORIZE FOR WEEK SIX:

*But you, man of God, flee from all this, and pursue righteousness, godliness, faith, love, endurance and gentleness.*

1 TIMOTHY 6:11

Date: _____

Name: _____

Home Phone: (_____) _____

Work Phone: (_____) _____

Email: _____

## Personal Prayer Concerns:

_____

_____

_____

_____

_____

_____

_____

This form is for prayer requests that are personal to you and your journey in First Place 4 Health. Please complete this form and have it ready to turn in when you arrive at your group meeting.

# First Place 4 Health
## Prayer Partner

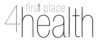

SCRIPTURE VERSE TO MEMORIZE FOR WEEK SEVEN:

*Do you not know that in a race all the runners run,*
*but only one gets the prize? Run in such a way as to get the prize.*

1 CORINTHIANS 9:24

Date: _____

Name: _____

Home Phone: (_____)_____

Work Phone: (_____)_____

Email: _____

**Personal Prayer Concerns:**

_____

_____

_____

_____

_____

_____

_____

This form is for prayer requests that are personal to you and your journey in First Place 4 Health. Please complete this form and have it ready to turn in when you arrive at your group meeting.

# First Place 4 Health
## Prayer Partner

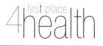

SCRIPTURE VERSE TO MEMORIZE FOR WEEK EIGHT:

*When the Chief Shepherd appears,*
*you will receive the crown of glory that will never fade away.*

1 PETER 5:4

Date: _____

Name: _____

Home Phone: ( ____ ) _____

Work Phone: ( ____ ) _____

Email: _____

**Personal Prayer Concerns:**

_____

_____

_____

_____

_____

_____

_____

This form is for prayer requests that are personal to you and your journey in First Place 4 Health. Please complete this form and have it ready to turn in when you arrive at your group meeting.

# First Place 4 Health
## Prayer Partner

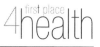

SCRIPTURE VERSE TO MEMORIZE FOR WEEK NINE:

*Therefore, since we are surrounded by such a great cloud of witnesses,*
*let us throw off everything that hinders and the sin that so easily entangles,*
*and let us run with perseverance the race marked out for us.*

HEBREWS 12:1

Date: _____

Name: _____

Home Phone: (_____) _____

Work Phone: (_____) _____

Email: _____

## Personal Prayer Concerns:

_____

_____

_____

_____

_____

_____

This form is for prayer requests that are personal to you and your journey in First Place 4 Health. Please complete this form and have it ready to turn in when you arrive at your group meeting.

# First Place 4 Health
## Prayer Partner

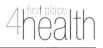

MOVING FORWARD
TOGETHER
Week
9

SCRIPTURE VERSE TO MEMORIZE FOR WEEK TEN:

*Let us fix our eyes on Jesus, the author and perfecter of our faith,*
*who for the joy set before him endured the cross, scorning its shame,*
*and sat down at the right hand of the throne of God.*

HEBREWS 12:2

Date: _____

Name: _____

Home Phone: (_____)_____

Work Phone: (_____)_____

Email: _____

## Personal Prayer Concerns:

_____

_____

_____

_____

_____

_____

_____

This form is for prayer requests that are personal to you and your journey in First Place 4 Health. Please complete this form and have it ready to turn in when you arrive at your group meeting.

*First Place 4 Health*
*Prayer Partner*

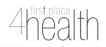

MOVING FORWARD
TOGETHER
**Week**
**10**

*See to it that no one misses the grace of God*
*and that no bitter root grows up to cause trouble and defile many.*

Hebrews 12:15

Date: _____

Name: _____

Home Phone: (_____)_____

Work Phone: (_____)_____

Email: _____

### Personal Prayer Concerns:

_____

_____

_____

_____

_____

_____

_____

This form is for prayer requests that are personal to you and your journey in First Place 4 Health. Please complete this form and have it ready to turn in when you arrive at your group meeting.

# First Place 4 Health
## Prayer Partner

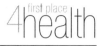

MOVING FORWARD
TOGETHER
Week
**11**

Date: _____

Name: _____

Home Phone: (_____) _____

Work Phone: (_____) _____

Email: _____

## Personal Prayer Concerns:

_____

_____

_____

_____

_____

_____

This form is for prayer requests that are personal to you and your journey in First Place 4 Health. Please complete this form and have it ready to turn in when you arrive at your group meeting.

# Live It Tracker

Name: _____    My week at a glance:  ❏ Great  ❏ So-so  ❏ Not so great

Date: _____ Week #: _____ Calorie Range: _____    My food goal for next week: _____

Activity Level:  None, < 30 min/day, 30-60 min/day, 60+ min/day    My activity goal for next week: _____

Scripture Memory Verse: _____

## RECOMMENDED DAILY AMOUNT OF FOOD FROM EACH GROUP

| Group | Daily Calories | | | | | | | |
|-------|-----------|-----------|-----------|-----------|-----------|-----------|-----------|-----------|
|       | 1300-1400 | 1500-1600 | 1700-1800 | 1900-2000 | 2100-2200 | 2300-2400 | 2500-2600 | 2700-2800 |
| Fruits | 1.5-2 c. | 1.5-2 c. | 1.5-2 c. | 2-2.5 c. | 2-2.5 c. | 2.5-3.5 c. | 3.5-4.5 c. | 3.5-4.5 c. |
| Vegetables | 1.5-2 c. | 2-2.5 c. | 2.5-3 c. | 2.5-3 c. | 3-3.5 c. | 3.5-4.5 c. | 4.5-5 c. | 4.5-5 c. |
| Grains | 5 oz-eq. | 5-6 oz-eq. | 6-7 oz-eq. | 6-7 oz-eq. | 7-8 oz-eq. | 8-9 oz-eq. | 9-10 oz-eq. | 10-11 oz-eq. |
| Meat & Beans | 4 oz-eq. | 5 oz-eq. | 5-5.5 oz-eq. | 5.5-6.5 oz-eq. | 6.5-7 oz-eq. | 7-7.5 oz-eq. | 7-7.5 oz-eq. | 7.5-8 oz-eq. |
| Milk | 2-3 c. | 3 c. | 3 c. | 3 c. | 3 c. | 3 c. | 3 c. | 3 c. |
| Healthy Oils | 4 tsp. | 5 tsp. | 5 tsp. | 6 tsp. | 6 tsp. | 7 tsp. | 8 tsp. | 8 tsp. |

### Day One

**FOOD CHOICES**

Breakfast: _____    Lunch: _____

Dinner: _____    Snacks: _____

| Group | Fruits | Vegetables | Grains | Meat & Beans | Milk | Oils |
|-------|--------|------------|--------|--------------|------|------|
| Goal Amount | | | | | | |
| Estimate Your Total | | | | | | |
| Increase ⇧ or Decrease ⇩ ? | | | | | | |

**PHYSICAL ACTIVITY**    **SPIRITUAL ACTIVITY**

Description: _____    Description: _____

Steps/Miles/Minutes: _____

### Day Two

**FOOD CHOICES**

Breakfast: _____    Lunch: _____

Dinner: _____    Snacks: _____

| Group | Fruits | Vegetables | Grains | Meat & Beans | Milk | Oils |
|-------|--------|------------|--------|--------------|------|------|
| Goal Amount | | | | | | |
| Estimate Your Total | | | | | | |
| Increase ⇧ or Decrease ⇩ ? | | | | | | |

**PHYSICAL ACTIVITY**    **SPIRITUAL ACTIVITY**

Description: _____    Description: _____

Steps/Miles/Minutes: _____

### Day Three

**FOOD CHOICES**

Breakfast: _____    Lunch: _____

Dinner: _____    Snacks: _____

| Group | Fruits | Vegetables | Grains | Meat & Beans | Milk | Oils |
|-------|--------|------------|--------|--------------|------|------|
| Goal Amount | | | | | | |
| Estimate Your Total | | | | | | |
| Increase ⇧ or Decrease ⇩ ? | | | | | | |

**PHYSICAL ACTIVITY**    **SPIRITUAL ACTIVITY**

Description: _____    Description: _____

Steps/Miles/Minutes: _____

## Day Four

**FOOD CHOICES**

Breakfast: _____  Lunch: _____

Dinner: _____  Snacks: _____

| Group | Fruits | Vegetables | Grains | Meat & Beans | Milk | Oils |
|---|---|---|---|---|---|---|
| Goal Amount | | | | | | |
| Estimate Your Total | | | | | | |
| Increase ⇧ or Decrease ⇩ ? | | | | | | |

**PHYSICAL ACTIVITY**

Description: _____

Steps/Miles/Minutes: _____

**SPIRITUAL ACTIVITY**

Description: _____

_____

## Day Five

**FOOD CHOICES**

Breakfast: _____  Lunch: _____

Dinner: _____  Snacks: _____

| Group | Fruits | Vegetables | Grains | Meat & Beans | Milk | Oils |
|---|---|---|---|---|---|---|
| Goal Amount | | | | | | |
| Estimate Your Total | | | | | | |
| Increase ⇧ or Decrease ⇩ ? | | | | | | |

**PHYSICAL ACTIVITY**

Description: _____

Steps/Miles/Minutes: _____

**SPIRITUAL ACTIVITY**

Description: _____

_____

## Day Six

**FOOD CHOICES**

Breakfast: _____  Lunch: _____

Dinner: _____  Snacks: _____

| Group | Fruits | Vegetables | Grains | Meat & Beans | Milk | Oils |
|---|---|---|---|---|---|---|
| Goal Amount | | | | | | |
| Estimate Your Total | | | | | | |
| Increase ⇧ or Decrease ⇩ ? | | | | | | |

**PHYSICAL ACTIVITY**

Description: _____

Steps/Miles/Minutes: _____

**SPIRITUAL ACTIVITY**

Description: _____

_____

## Day Seven

**FOOD CHOICES**

Breakfast: _____  Lunch: _____

Dinner: _____  Snacks: _____

| Group | Fruits | Vegetables | Grains | Meat & Beans | Milk | Oils |
|---|---|---|---|---|---|---|
| Goal Amount | | | | | | |
| Estimate Your Total | | | | | | |
| Increase ⇧ or Decrease ⇩ ? | | | | | | |

**PHYSICAL ACTIVITY**

Description: _____

Steps/Miles/Minutes: _____

**SPIRITUAL ACTIVITY**

Description: _____

_____

# Live It Tracker

Name: _____    My week at a glance: ☐ Great ☐ So-so ☐ Not so great

Date: _____ Week #: _____ Calorie Range: _____    My food goal for next week: _____

Activity Level: None, < 30 min/day, 30-60 min/day, 60+ min/day    My activity goal for next week: _____

Scripture Memory Verse: _____

## RECOMMENDED DAILY AMOUNT OF FOOD FROM EACH GROUP

| Group | Daily Calories | | | | | | | |
|---|---|---|---|---|---|---|---|---|
| | 1300-1400 | 1500-1600 | 1700-1800 | 1900-2000 | 2100-2200 | 2300-2400 | 2500-2600 | 2700-2800 |
| Fruits | 1.5-2 c. | 1.5-2 c. | 1.5-2 c. | 2-2.5 c. | 2-2.5 c. | 2.5-3.5 c. | 3.5-4.5 c. | 3.5-4.5 c. |
| Vegetables | 1.5-2 c. | 2-2.5 c. | 2.5-3 c. | 2.5-3 c. | 3-3.5 c. | 3.5-4.5 c. | 4.5-5 c. | 4.5-5 c. |
| Grains | 5 oz-eq. | 5-6 oz-eq. | 6-7 oz-eq. | 6-7 oz-eq. | 7-8 oz-eq. | 8-9 oz-eq. | 9-10 oz-eq. | 10-11 oz-eq. |
| Meat & Beans | 4 oz-eq. | 5 oz-eq. | 5-5.5 oz-eq. | 5.5-6.5 oz-eq. | 6.5-7 oz-eq. | 7-7.5 oz-eq. | 7-7.5 oz-eq. | 7.5-8 oz-eq. |
| Milk | 2-3 c. | 3 c. | 3 c. | 3 c. | 3 c. | 3 c. | 3 c. | 3 c. |
| Healthy Oils | 4 tsp. | 5 tsp. | 5 tsp. | 6 tsp. | 6 tsp. | 7 tsp. | 8 tsp. | 8 tsp. |

## Day One

### FOOD CHOICES

Breakfast: _____    Lunch: _____

Dinner: _____    Snacks: _____

| Group | Fruits | Vegetables | Grains | Meat & Beans | Milk | Oils |
|---|---|---|---|---|---|---|
| Goal Amount | | | | | | |
| Estimate Your Total | | | | | | |
| Increase ⇧ or Decrease ⇩ ? | | | | | | |

### PHYSICAL ACTIVITY

Description: _____

Steps/Miles/Minutes: _____

### SPIRITUAL ACTIVITY

Description: _____

_____

## Day Two

### FOOD CHOICES

Breakfast: _____    Lunch: _____

Dinner: _____    Snacks: _____

| Group | Fruits | Vegetables | Grains | Meat & Beans | Milk | Oils |
|---|---|---|---|---|---|---|
| Goal Amount | | | | | | |
| Estimate Your Total | | | | | | |
| Increase ⇧ or Decrease ⇩ ? | | | | | | |

### PHYSICAL ACTIVITY

Description: _____

Steps/Miles/Minutes: _____

### SPIRITUAL ACTIVITY

Description: _____

_____

## Day Three

### FOOD CHOICES

Breakfast: _____    Lunch: _____

Dinner: _____    Snacks: _____

| Group | Fruits | Vegetables | Grains | Meat & Beans | Milk | Oils |
|---|---|---|---|---|---|---|
| Goal Amount | | | | | | |
| Estimate Your Total | | | | | | |
| Increase ⇧ or Decrease ⇩ ? | | | | | | |

### PHYSICAL ACTIVITY

Description: _____

Steps/Miles/Minutes: _____

### SPIRITUAL ACTIVITY

Description: _____

_____

## FOOD CHOICES

Breakfast: _____    Lunch: _____

Dinner: _____    Snacks: _____

| Group | Fruits | Vegetables | Grains | Meat & Beans | Milk | Oils |
|---|---|---|---|---|---|---|
| Goal Amount | | | | | | |
| Estimate Your Total | | | | | | |
| Increase ⇧ or Decrease ⇩ ? | | | | | | |

### PHYSICAL ACTIVITY

Description: _____

Steps/Miles/Minutes: _____

### SPIRITUAL ACTIVITY

Description: _____

_____

## FOOD CHOICES

Breakfast: _____    Lunch: _____

Dinner: _____    Snacks: _____

| Group | Fruits | Vegetables | Grains | Meat & Beans | Milk | Oils |
|---|---|---|---|---|---|---|
| Goal Amount | | | | | | |
| Estimate Your Total | | | | | | |
| Increase ⇧ or Decrease ⇩ ? | | | | | | |

### PHYSICAL ACTIVITY

Description: _____

Steps/Miles/Minutes: _____

### SPIRITUAL ACTIVITY

Description: _____

_____

## FOOD CHOICES

Breakfast: _____    Lunch: _____

Dinner: _____    Snacks: _____

| Group | Fruits | Vegetables | Grains | Meat & Beans | Milk | Oils |
|---|---|---|---|---|---|---|
| Goal Amount | | | | | | |
| Estimate Your Total | | | | | | |
| Increase ⇧ or Decrease ⇩ ? | | | | | | |

### PHYSICAL ACTIVITY

Description: _____

Steps/Miles/Minutes: _____

### SPIRITUAL ACTIVITY

Description: _____

_____

## FOOD CHOICES

Breakfast: _____    Lunch: _____

Dinner: _____    Snacks: _____

| Group | Fruits | Vegetables | Grains | Meat & Beans | Milk | Oils |
|---|---|---|---|---|---|---|
| Goal Amount | | | | | | |
| Estimate Your Total | | | | | | |
| Increase ⇧ or Decrease ⇩ ? | | | | | | |

### PHYSICAL ACTIVITY

Description: _____

Steps/Miles/Minutes: _____

### SPIRITUAL ACTIVITY

Description: _____

_____

# Live It Tracker

Name: _____

My week at a glance: ❑ Great  ❑ So-so  ❑ Not so great

Date: _____ Week #: _____ Calorie Range: _____

My food goal for next week: _____

Activity Level: None, < 30 min/day, 30-60 min/day, 60+ min/day

My activity goal for next week: _____

Scripture Memory Verse: _____

## RECOMMENDED DAILY AMOUNT OF FOOD FROM EACH GROUP

| Group | Daily Calories | | | | | | | |
|---|---|---|---|---|---|---|---|---|
| | 1300-1400 | 1500-1600 | 1700-1800 | 1900-2000 | 2100-2200 | 2300-2400 | 2500-2600 | 2700-2800 |
| Fruits | 1.5-2 c. | 1.5-2 c. | 1.5-2 c. | 2-2.5 c. | 2-2.5 c. | 2.5-3.5 c. | 3.5-4.5 c. | 3.5-4.5 c. |
| Vegetables | 1.5-2 c. | 2-2.5 c. | 2.5-3 c. | 2.5-3 c. | 3-3.5 c. | 3.5-4.5 c. | 4.5-5 c. | 4.5-5 c. |
| Grains | 5 oz-eq. | 5-6 oz-eq. | 6-7 oz-eq. | 6-7 oz-eq. | 7-8 oz-eq. | 8-9 oz-eq. | 9-10 oz-eq. | 10-11 oz-eq. |
| Meat & Beans | 4 oz-eq. | 5 oz-eq. | 5-5.5 oz-eq. | 5.5-6.5 oz-eq. | 6.5-7 oz-eq. | 7-7.5 oz-eq. | 7-7.5 oz-eq. | 7.5-8 oz-eq. |
| Milk | 2-3 c. | 3 c. | 3 c. | 3 c. | 3 c. | 3 c. | 3 c. | 3 c. |
| Healthy Oils | 4 tsp. | 5 tsp. | 5 tsp. | 6 tsp. | 6 tsp. | 7 tsp. | 8 tsp. | 8 tsp. |

## Day One

### FOOD CHOICES

Breakfast: _____  Lunch: _____

Dinner: _____  Snacks: _____

| Group | Fruits | Vegetables | Grains | Meat & Beans | Milk | Oils |
|---|---|---|---|---|---|---|
| Goal Amount | | | | | | |
| Estimate Your Total | | | | | | |
| Increase ⬆ or Decrease ⬇ ? | | | | | | |

### PHYSICAL ACTIVITY

Description: _____

Steps/Miles/Minutes: _____

### SPIRITUAL ACTIVITY

Description: _____

_____

## Day Two

### FOOD CHOICES

Breakfast: _____  Lunch: _____

Dinner: _____  Snacks: _____

| Group | Fruits | Vegetables | Grains | Meat & Beans | Milk | Oils |
|---|---|---|---|---|---|---|
| Goal Amount | | | | | | |
| Estimate Your Total | | | | | | |
| Increase ⬆ or Decrease ⬇ ? | | | | | | |

### PHYSICAL ACTIVITY

Description: _____

Steps/Miles/Minutes: _____

### SPIRITUAL ACTIVITY

Description: _____

_____

## Day Three

### FOOD CHOICES

Breakfast: _____  Lunch: _____

Dinner: _____  Snacks: _____

| Group | Fruits | Vegetables | Grains | Meat & Beans | Milk | Oils |
|---|---|---|---|---|---|---|
| Goal Amount | | | | | | |
| Estimate Your Total | | | | | | |
| Increase ⬆ or Decrease ⬇ ? | | | | | | |

### PHYSICAL ACTIVITY

Description: _____

Steps/Miles/Minutes: _____

### SPIRITUAL ACTIVITY

Description: _____

_____

## Day Four

### FOOD CHOICES

Breakfast: _____   Lunch: _____

Dinner: _____   Snacks: _____

| Group | Fruits | Vegetables | Grains | Meat & Beans | Milk | Oils |
|---|---|---|---|---|---|---|
| Goal Amount | | | | | | |
| Estimate Your Total | | | | | | |
| Increase ⇧ or Decrease ⇩ ? | | | | | | |

### PHYSICAL ACTIVITY

Description: _____

Steps/Miles/Minutes: _____

### SPIRITUAL ACTIVITY

Description: _____

_____

## Day Five

### FOOD CHOICES

Breakfast: _____   Lunch: _____

Dinner: _____   Snacks: _____

| Group | Fruits | Vegetables | Grains | Meat & Beans | Milk | Oils |
|---|---|---|---|---|---|---|
| Goal Amount | | | | | | |
| Estimate Your Total | | | | | | |
| Increase ⇧ or Decrease ⇩ ? | | | | | | |

### PHYSICAL ACTIVITY

Description: _____

Steps/Miles/Minutes: _____

### SPIRITUAL ACTIVITY

Description: _____

_____

## Day Six

### FOOD CHOICES

Breakfast: _____   Lunch: _____

Dinner: _____   Snacks: _____

| Group | Fruits | Vegetables | Grains | Meat & Beans | Milk | Oils |
|---|---|---|---|---|---|---|
| Goal Amount | | | | | | |
| Estimate Your Total | | | | | | |
| Increase ⇧ or Decrease ⇩ ? | | | | | | |

### PHYSICAL ACTIVITY

Description: _____

Steps/Miles/Minutes: _____

### SPIRITUAL ACTIVITY

Description: _____

_____

## Day Seven

### FOOD CHOICES

Breakfast: _____   Lunch: _____

Dinner: _____   Snacks: _____

| Group | Fruits | Vegetables | Grains | Meat & Beans | Milk | Oils |
|---|---|---|---|---|---|---|
| Goal Amount | | | | | | |
| Estimate Your Total | | | | | | |
| Increase ⇧ or Decrease ⇩ ? | | | | | | |

### PHYSICAL ACTIVITY

Description: _____

Steps/Miles/Minutes: _____

### SPIRITUAL ACTIVITY

Description: _____

_____

# Live It Tracker

Name: _____     My week at a glance: ☐ Great  ☐ So-so  ☐ Not so great

Date: _____ Week #: _____ Calorie Range: _____     My food goal for next week: _____

Activity Level: None, < 30 min/day, 30-60 min/day, 60+ min/day   My activity goal for next week: _____

Scripture Memory Verse: _____

## RECOMMENDED DAILY AMOUNT OF FOOD FROM EACH GROUP

| Group | Daily Calories | | | | | | | |
|---|---|---|---|---|---|---|---|---|
| | 1300-1400 | 1500-1600 | 1700-1800 | 1900-2000 | 2100-2200 | 2300-2400 | 2500-2600 | 2700-2800 |
| Fruits | 1.5-2 c. | 1.5-2 c. | 1.5-2 c. | 2-2.5 c. | 2-2.5 c. | 2.5-3.5 c. | 3.5-4.5 c. | 3.5-4.5 c. |
| Vegetables | 1.5-2 c. | 2-2.5 c. | 2.5-3 c. | 2.5-3 c. | 3-3.5 c. | 3.5-4.5 c. | 4.5-5 c. | 4.5-5 c. |
| Grains | 5 oz-eq. | 5-6 oz-eq. | 6-7 oz-eq. | 6-7 oz-eq. | 7-8 oz-eq. | 8-9 oz-eq. | 9-10 oz-eq. | 10-11 oz-eq. |
| Meat & Beans | 4 oz-eq. | 5 oz-eq. | 5-5.5 oz-eq. | 5.5-6.5 oz-eq. | 6.5-7 oz-eq. | 7-7.5 oz-eq. | 7-7.5 oz-eq. | 7.5-8 oz-eq. |
| Milk | 2-3 c. | 3 c. | 3 c. | 3 c. | 3 c. | 3 c. | 3 c. | 3 c. |
| Healthy Oils | 4 tsp. | 5 tsp. | 5 tsp. | 6 tsp. | 6 tsp. | 7 tsp. | 8 tsp. | 8 tsp. |

## FOOD CHOICES

Breakfast: _____     Lunch: _____

Dinner: _____     Snacks: _____

**Day One**

| Group | Fruits | Vegetables | Grains | Meat & Beans | Milk | Oils |
|---|---|---|---|---|---|---|
| Goal Amount | | | | | | |
| Estimate Your Total | | | | | | |
| Increase ⇧ or Decrease ⇩ ? | | | | | | |

### PHYSICAL ACTIVITY
Description: _____

Steps/Miles/Minutes: _____

### SPIRITUAL ACTIVITY
Description: _____

_____

## FOOD CHOICES

Breakfast: _____     Lunch: _____

Dinner: _____     Snacks: _____

**Day Two**

| Group | Fruits | Vegetables | Grains | Meat & Beans | Milk | Oils |
|---|---|---|---|---|---|---|
| Goal Amount | | | | | | |
| Estimate Your Total | | | | | | |
| Increase ⇧ or Decrease ⇩ ? | | | | | | |

### PHYSICAL ACTIVITY
Description: _____

Steps/Miles/Minutes: _____

### SPIRITUAL ACTIVITY
Description: _____

_____

## FOOD CHOICES

Breakfast: _____     Lunch: _____

Dinner: _____     Snacks: _____

**Day Three**

| Group | Fruits | Vegetables | Grains | Meat & Beans | Milk | Oils |
|---|---|---|---|---|---|---|
| Goal Amount | | | | | | |
| Estimate Your Total | | | | | | |
| Increase ⇧ or Decrease ⇩ ? | | | | | | |

### PHYSICAL ACTIVITY
Description: _____

Steps/Miles/Minutes: _____

### SPIRITUAL ACTIVITY
Description: _____

## Day Four

FOOD CHOICES

Breakfast: _____  Lunch: _____

Dinner: _____  Snacks: _____

| Group | Fruits | Vegetables | Grains | Meat & Beans | Milk | Oils |
|---|---|---|---|---|---|---|
| Goal Amount | | | | | | |
| Estimate Your Total | | | | | | |
| Increase ⬆ or Decrease ⬇ ? | | | | | | |

PHYSICAL ACTIVITY

Description: _____

Steps/Miles/Minutes: _____

SPIRITUAL ACTIVITY

Description: _____

---

## Day Five

FOOD CHOICES

Breakfast: _____  Lunch: _____

Dinner: _____  Snacks: _____

| Group | Fruits | Vegetables | Grains | Meat & Beans | Milk | Oils |
|---|---|---|---|---|---|---|
| Goal Amount | | | | | | |
| Estimate Your Total | | | | | | |
| Increase ⬆ or Decrease ⬇ ? | | | | | | |

PHYSICAL ACTIVITY

Description: _____

Steps/Miles/Minutes: _____

SPIRITUAL ACTIVITY

Description: _____

---

## Day Six

FOOD CHOICES

Breakfast: _____  Lunch: _____

Dinner: _____  Snacks: _____

| Group | Fruits | Vegetables | Grains | Meat & Beans | Milk | Oils |
|---|---|---|---|---|---|---|
| Goal Amount | | | | | | |
| Estimate Your Total | | | | | | |
| Increase ⬆ or Decrease ⬇ ? | | | | | | |

PHYSICAL ACTIVITY

Description: _____

Steps/Miles/Minutes: _____

SPIRITUAL ACTIVITY

Description: _____

---

## Day Seven

FOOD CHOICES

Breakfast: _____  Lunch: _____

Dinner: _____  Snacks: _____

| Group | Fruits | Vegetables | Grains | Meat & Beans | Milk | Oils |
|---|---|---|---|---|---|---|
| Goal Amount | | | | | | |
| Estimate Your Total | | | | | | |
| Increase ⬆ or Decrease ⬇ ? | | | | | | |

PHYSICAL ACTIVITY

Description: _____

Steps/Miles/Minutes: _____

SPIRITUAL ACTIVITY

Description: _____

# Live It Tracker

Name: _____  My week at a glance: ☐ Great ☐ So-so ☐ Not so great

Date: _____ Week #: _____ Calorie Range: _____  My food goal for next week: _____

Activity Level: None, < 30 min/day, 30-60 min/day, 60+ min/day  My activity goal for next week: _____

Scripture Memory Verse: _____

RECOMMENDED DAILY AMOUNT OF FOOD FROM EACH GROUP

| Group | Daily Calories | | | | | | | |
|---|---|---|---|---|---|---|---|---|
| | 1300-1400 | 1500-1600 | 1700-1800 | 1900-2000 | 2100-2200 | 2300-2400 | 2500-2600 | 2700-2800 |
| Fruits | 1.5-2 c. | 1.5-2 c. | 1.5-2 c. | 2-2.5 c. | 2-2.5 c. | 2.5-3.5 c. | 3.5-4.5 c. | 3.5-4.5 c. |
| Vegetables | 1.5-2 c. | 2-2.5 c. | 2.5-3 c. | 2.5-3 c. | 3-3.5 c. | 3.5-4.5 c. | 4.5-5 c. | 4.5-5 c. |
| Grains | 5 oz-eq. | 5-6 oz-eq. | 6-7 oz-eq. | 6-7 oz-eq. | 7-8 oz-eq. | 8-9 oz-eq. | 9-10 oz-eq. | 10-11 oz-eq. |
| Meat & Beans | 4 oz-eq. | 5 oz-eq. | 5-5.5 oz-eq. | 5.5-6.5 oz-eq. | 6.5-7 oz-eq. | 7-7.5 oz-eq. | 7-7.5 oz-eq. | 7.5-8 oz-eq. |
| Milk | 2-3 c. | 3 c. | 3 c. | 3 c. | 3 c. | 3 c. | 3 c. | 3 c. |
| Healthy Oils | 4 tsp. | 5 tsp. | 5 tsp. | 6 tsp. | 6 tsp. | 7 tsp. | 8 tsp. | 8 tsp. |

## Day One

**FOOD CHOICES**

Breakfast: _____  Lunch: _____

Dinner: _____  Snacks: _____

| Group | Fruits | Vegetables | Grains | Meat & Beans | Milk | Oils |
|---|---|---|---|---|---|---|
| Goal Amount | | | | | | |
| Estimate Your Total | | | | | | |
| Increase ⇧ or Decrease ⇩ ? | | | | | | |

**PHYSICAL ACTIVITY**

Description: _____

Steps/Miles/Minutes: _____

**SPIRITUAL ACTIVITY**

Description: _____

_____

## Day Two

**FOOD CHOICES**

Breakfast: _____  Lunch: _____

Dinner: _____  Snacks: _____

| Group | Fruits | Vegetables | Grains | Meat & Beans | Milk | Oils |
|---|---|---|---|---|---|---|
| Goal Amount | | | | | | |
| Estimate Your Total | | | | | | |
| Increase ⇧ or Decrease ⇩ ? | | | | | | |

**PHYSICAL ACTIVITY**

Description: _____

Steps/Miles/Minutes: _____

**SPIRITUAL ACTIVITY**

Description: _____

_____

## Day Three

**FOOD CHOICES**

Breakfast: _____  Lunch: _____

Dinner: _____  Snacks: _____

| Group | Fruits | Vegetables | Grains | Meat & Beans | Milk | Oils |
|---|---|---|---|---|---|---|
| Goal Amount | | | | | | |
| Estimate Your Total | | | | | | |
| Increase ⇧ or Decrease ⇩ ? | | | | | | |

**PHYSICAL ACTIVITY**

Description: _____

Steps/Miles/Minutes: _____

**SPIRITUAL ACTIVITY**

Description: _____

_____

## Day Four

### FOOD CHOICES

Breakfast: _____  Lunch: _____

Dinner: _____  Snacks: _____

| Group | Fruits | Vegetables | Grains | Meat & Beans | Milk | Oils |
|---|---|---|---|---|---|---|
| Goal Amount | | | | | | |
| Estimate Your Total | | | | | | |
| Increase ⇧ or Decrease ⇩ ? | | | | | | |

### PHYSICAL ACTIVITY

Description: _____

Steps/Miles/Minutes: _____

### SPIRITUAL ACTIVITY

Description: _____

_____

## Day Five

### FOOD CHOICES

Breakfast: _____  Lunch: _____

Dinner: _____  Snacks: _____

| Group | Fruits | Vegetables | Grains | Meat & Beans | Milk | Oils |
|---|---|---|---|---|---|---|
| Goal Amount | | | | | | |
| Estimate Your Total | | | | | | |
| Increase ⇧ or Decrease ⇩ ? | | | | | | |

### PHYSICAL ACTIVITY

Description: _____

Steps/Miles/Minutes: _____

### SPIRITUAL ACTIVITY

Description: _____

_____

## Day Six

### FOOD CHOICES

Breakfast: _____  Lunch: _____

Dinner: _____  Snacks: _____

| Group | Fruits | Vegetables | Grains | Meat & Beans | Milk | Oils |
|---|---|---|---|---|---|---|
| Goal Amount | | | | | | |
| Estimate Your Total | | | | | | |
| Increase ⇧ or Decrease ⇩ ? | | | | | | |

### PHYSICAL ACTIVITY

Description: _____

Steps/Miles/Minutes: _____

### SPIRITUAL ACTIVITY

Description: _____

_____

## Day Seven

### FOOD CHOICES

Breakfast: _____  Lunch: _____

Dinner: _____  Snacks: _____

| Group | Fruits | Vegetables | Grains | Meat & Beans | Milk | Oils |
|---|---|---|---|---|---|---|
| Goal Amount | | | | | | |
| Estimate Your Total | | | | | | |
| Increase ⇧ or Decrease ⇩ ? | | | | | | |

### PHYSICAL ACTIVITY

Description: _____

Steps/Miles/Minutes: _____

### SPIRITUAL ACTIVITY

Description: _____

_____

# Live It Tracker

Name: _____  My week at a glance: ❏ Great  ❏ So-so  ❏ Not so great

Date: _____ Week #: _____ Calorie Range: _____  My food goal for next week: _____

Activity Level: None, < 30 min/day, 30-60 min/day, 60+ min/day  My activity goal for next week: _____

Scripture Memory Verse: _____

## RECOMMENDED DAILY AMOUNT OF FOOD FROM EACH GROUP

| Group | Daily Calories | | | | | | | |
|---|---|---|---|---|---|---|---|---|
| | 1300-1400 | 1500-1600 | 1700-1800 | 1900-2000 | 2100-2200 | 2300-2400 | 2500-2600 | 2700-2800 |
| Fruits | 1.5-2 c. | 1.5-2 c. | 1.5-2 c. | 2-2.5 c. | 2-2.5 c. | 2.5-3.5 c. | 3.5-4.5 c. | 3.5-4.5 c. |
| Vegetables | 1.5-2 c. | 2-2.5 c. | 2.5-3 c. | 2.5-3 c. | 3-3.5 c. | 3.5-4.5 c. | 4.5-5 c. | 4.5-5 c. |
| Grains | 5 oz-eq. | 5-6 oz-eq. | 6-7 oz-eq. | 6-7 oz-eq. | 7-8 oz-eq. | 8-9 oz-eq. | 9-10 oz-eq. | 10-11 oz-eq. |
| Meat & Beans | 4 oz-eq. | 5 oz-eq. | 5-5.5 oz-eq. | 5.5-6.5 oz-eq. | 6.5-7 oz-eq. | 7-7.5 oz-eq. | 7-7.5 oz-eq. | 7.5-8 oz-eq. |
| Milk | 2-3 c. | 3 c. | 3 c. | 3 c. | 3 c. | 3 c. | 3 c. | 3 c. |
| Healthy Oils | 4 tsp. | 5 tsp. | 5 tsp. | 6 tsp. | 6 tsp. | 7 tsp. | 8 tsp. | 8 tsp. |

### Day One

**FOOD CHOICES**

Breakfast: _____  Lunch: _____

Dinner: _____  Snacks: _____

| Group | Fruits | Vegetables | Grains | Meat & Beans | Milk | Oils |
|---|---|---|---|---|---|---|
| Goal Amount | | | | | | |
| Estimate Your Total | | | | | | |
| Increase ⇧ or Decrease ⇩ ? | | | | | | |

**PHYSICAL ACTIVITY**

Description: _____

Steps/Miles/Minutes: _____

**SPIRITUAL ACTIVITY**

Description: _____

_____

### Day Two

**FOOD CHOICES**

Breakfast: _____  Lunch: _____

Dinner: _____  Snacks: _____

| Group | Fruits | Vegetables | Grains | Meat & Beans | Milk | Oils |
|---|---|---|---|---|---|---|
| Goal Amount | | | | | | |
| Estimate Your Total | | | | | | |
| Increase ⇧ or Decrease ⇩ ? | | | | | | |

**PHYSICAL ACTIVITY**

Description: _____

Steps/Miles/Minutes: _____

**SPIRITUAL ACTIVITY**

Description: _____

_____

### Day Three

**FOOD CHOICES**

Breakfast: _____  Lunch: _____

Dinner: _____  Snacks: _____

| Group | Fruits | Vegetables | Grains | Meat & Beans | Milk | Oils |
|---|---|---|---|---|---|---|
| Goal Amount | | | | | | |
| Estimate Your Total | | | | | | |
| Increase ⇧ or Decrease ⇩ ? | | | | | | |

**PHYSICAL ACTIVITY**

Description: _____

Steps/Miles/Minutes: _____

**SPIRITUAL ACTIVITY**

Description: _____

_____

## FOOD CHOICES

Breakfast: _____    Lunch: _____

Dinner: _____    Snacks: _____

| Group | Fruits | Vegetables | Grains | Meat & Beans | Milk | Oils |
|---|---|---|---|---|---|---|
| Goal Amount | | | | | | |
| Estimate Your Total | | | | | | |
| Increase ⇧ or Decrease ⇩ ? | | | | | | |

### PHYSICAL ACTIVITY

Description: _____

Steps/Miles/Minutes: _____

### SPIRITUAL ACTIVITY

Description: _____

_____

## FOOD CHOICES

Breakfast: _____    Lunch: _____

Dinner: _____    Snacks: _____

| Group | Fruits | Vegetables | Grains | Meat & Beans | Milk | Oils |
|---|---|---|---|---|---|---|
| Goal Amount | | | | | | |
| Estimate Your Total | | | | | | |
| Increase ⇧ or Decrease ⇩ ? | | | | | | |

### PHYSICAL ACTIVITY

Description: _____

Steps/Miles/Minutes: _____

### SPIRITUAL ACTIVITY

Description: _____

_____

## FOOD CHOICES

Breakfast: _____    Lunch: _____

Dinner: _____    Snacks: _____

| Group | Fruits | Vegetables | Grains | Meat & Beans | Milk | Oils |
|---|---|---|---|---|---|---|
| Goal Amount | | | | | | |
| Estimate Your Total | | | | | | |
| Increase ⇧ or Decrease ⇩ ? | | | | | | |

### PHYSICAL ACTIVITY

Description: _____

Steps/Miles/Minutes: _____

### SPIRITUAL ACTIVITY

Description: _____

_____

## FOOD CHOICES

Breakfast: _____    Lunch: _____

Dinner: _____    Snacks: _____

| Group | Fruits | Vegetables | Grains | Meat & Beans | Milk | Oils |
|---|---|---|---|---|---|---|
| Goal Amount | | | | | | |
| Estimate Your Total | | | | | | |
| Increase ⇧ or Decrease ⇩ ? | | | | | | |

### PHYSICAL ACTIVITY

Description: _____

Steps/Miles/Minutes: _____

### SPIRITUAL ACTIVITY

Description: _____

_____

# Live It Tracker

Name: _____ My week at a glance: ❑ Great ❑ So-so ❑ Not so great

Date: _____ Week #: _____ Calorie Range: _____ My food goal for next week: _____

Activity Level: None, < 30 min/day, 30-60 min/day, 60+ min/day   My activity goal for next week: _____

Scripture Memory Verse: _____

## RECOMMENDED DAILY AMOUNT OF FOOD FROM EACH GROUP

| Group | Daily Calories | | | | | | | |
|-------|-----------|-----------|-----------|-----------|-----------|-----------|-----------|-----------|
|       | 1300-1400 | 1500-1600 | 1700-1800 | 1900-2000 | 2100-2200 | 2300-2400 | 2500-2600 | 2700-2800 |
| Fruits | 1.5-2 c. | 1.5-2 c. | 1.5-2 c. | 2-2.5 c. | 2-2.5 c. | 2.5-3.5 c. | 3.5-4.5 c. | 3.5-4.5 c. |
| Vegetables | 1.5-2 c. | 2-2.5 c. | 2.5-3 c. | 2.5-3 c. | 3-3.5 c. | 3.5-4.5 c. | 4.5-5 c. | 4.5-5 c. |
| Grains | 5 oz-eq. | 5-6 oz-eq. | 6-7 oz-eq. | 6-7 oz-eq. | 7-8 oz-eq. | 8-9 oz-eq. | 9-10 oz-eq. | 10-11 oz-eq. |
| Meat & Beans | 4 oz-eq. | 5 oz-eq. | 5-5.5 oz-eq. | 5.5-6.5 oz-eq. | 6.5-7 oz-eq. | 7-7.5 oz-eq. | 7-7.5 oz-eq. | 7.5-8 oz-eq. |
| Milk | 2-3 c. | 3 c. | 3 c. | 3 c. | 3 c. | 3 c. | 3 c. | 3 c. |
| Healthy Oils | 4 tsp. | 5 tsp. | 5 tsp. | 6 tsp. | 6 tsp. | 7 tsp. | 8 tsp. | 8 tsp. |

### FOOD CHOICES

Breakfast: _____ Lunch: _____

Dinner: _____ Snacks: _____

**Day One**

| Group | Fruits | Vegetables | Grains | Meat & Beans | Milk | Oils |
|-------|--------|------------|--------|--------------|------|------|
| Goal Amount | | | | | | |
| Estimate Your Total | | | | | | |
| Increase ⬆ or Decrease ⬇ ? | | | | | | |

PHYSICAL ACTIVITY

Description: _____

Steps/Miles/Minutes: _____

SPIRITUAL ACTIVITY

Description: _____

_____

### FOOD CHOICES

Breakfast: _____ Lunch: _____

Dinner: _____ Snacks: _____

**Day Two**

| Group | Fruits | Vegetables | Grains | Meat & Beans | Milk | Oils |
|-------|--------|------------|--------|--------------|------|------|
| Goal Amount | | | | | | |
| Estimate Your Total | | | | | | |
| Increase ⬆ or Decrease ⬇ ? | | | | | | |

PHYSICAL ACTIVITY

Description: _____

Steps/Miles/Minutes: _____

SPIRITUAL ACTIVITY

Description: _____

_____

### FOOD CHOICES

Breakfast: _____ Lunch: _____

Dinner: _____ Snacks: _____

**Day Three**

| Group | Fruits | Vegetables | Grains | Meat & Beans | Milk | Oils |
|-------|--------|------------|--------|--------------|------|------|
| Goal Amount | | | | | | |
| Estimate Your Total | | | | | | |
| Increase ⬆ or Decrease ⬇ ? | | | | | | |

PHYSICAL ACTIVITY

Description: _____

Steps/Miles/Minutes: _____

SPIRITUAL ACTIVITY

Description: _____

_____

## Day Four

### FOOD CHOICES

Breakfast: _____  Lunch: _____

Dinner: _____  Snacks: _____

| Group | Fruits | Vegetables | Grains | Meat & Beans | Milk | Oils |
|---|---|---|---|---|---|---|
| Goal Amount | | | | | | |
| Estimate Your Total | | | | | | |
| Increase ⇧ or Decrease ⇩ ? | | | | | | |

### PHYSICAL ACTIVITY

Description: _____

Steps/Miles/Minutes: _____

### SPIRITUAL ACTIVITY

Description: _____

_____

## Day Five

### FOOD CHOICES

Breakfast: _____  Lunch: _____

Dinner: _____  Snacks: _____

| Group | Fruits | Vegetables | Grains | Meat & Beans | Milk | Oils |
|---|---|---|---|---|---|---|
| Goal Amount | | | | | | |
| Estimate Your Total | | | | | | |
| Increase ⇧ or Decrease ⇩ ? | | | | | | |

### PHYSICAL ACTIVITY

Description: _____

Steps/Miles/Minutes: _____

### SPIRITUAL ACTIVITY

Description: _____

_____

## Day Six

### FOOD CHOICES

Breakfast: _____  Lunch: _____

Dinner: _____  Snacks: _____

| Group | Fruits | Vegetables | Grains | Meat & Beans | Milk | Oils |
|---|---|---|---|---|---|---|
| Goal Amount | | | | | | |
| Estimate Your Total | | | | | | |
| Increase ⇧ or Decrease ⇩ ? | | | | | | |

### PHYSICAL ACTIVITY

Description: _____

Steps/Miles/Minutes: _____

### SPIRITUAL ACTIVITY

Description: _____

_____

## Day Seven

### FOOD CHOICES

Breakfast: _____  Lunch: _____

Dinner: _____  Snacks: _____

| Group | Fruits | Vegetables | Grains | Meat & Beans | Milk | Oils |
|---|---|---|---|---|---|---|
| Goal Amount | | | | | | |
| Estimate Your Total | | | | | | |
| Increase ⇧ or Decrease ⇩ ? | | | | | | |

### PHYSICAL ACTIVITY

Description: _____

Steps/Miles/Minutes: _____

### SPIRITUAL ACTIVITY

Description: _____

_____

# Live It Tracker

Name: _____  My week at a glance: ☐ Great ☐ So-so ☐ Not so great

Date: _____ Week #: _____ Calorie Range: _____  My food goal for next week: _____

Activity Level: None, < 30 min/day, 30-60 min/day, 60+ min/day  My activity goal for next week: _____

Scripture Memory Verse: _____

## RECOMMENDED DAILY AMOUNT OF FOOD FROM EACH GROUP

| Group | Daily Calories | | | | | | | |
|-------|-----------|-----------|-----------|-----------|-----------|-----------|-----------|-----------|
| | 1300-1400 | 1500-1600 | 1700-1800 | 1900-2000 | 2100-2200 | 2300-2400 | 2500-2600 | 2700-2800 |
| Fruits | 1.5-2 c. | 1.5-2 c. | 1.5-2 c. | 2-2.5 c. | 2-2.5 c. | 2.5-3.5 c. | 3.5-4.5 c. | 3.5-4.5 c. |
| Vegetables | 1.5-2 c. | 2-2.5 c. | 2.5-3 c. | 2.5-3 c. | 3-3.5 c. | 3.5-4.5 c. | 4.5-5 c. | 4.5-5 c. |
| Grains | 5 oz-eq. | 5-6 oz-eq. | 6-7 oz-eq. | 6-7 oz-eq. | 7-8 oz-eq. | 8-9 oz-eq. | 9-10 oz-eq. | 10-11 oz-eq. |
| Meat & Beans | 4 oz-eq. | 5 oz-eq. | 5-5.5 oz-eq. | 5.5-6.5 oz-eq. | 6.5-7 oz-eq. | 7-7.5 oz-eq. | 7-7.5 oz-eq. | 7.5-8 oz-eq. |
| Milk | 2-3 c. | 3 c. | 3 c. | 3 c. | 3 c. | 3 c. | 3 c. | 3 c. |
| Healthy Oils | 4 tsp. | 5 tsp. | 5 tsp. | 6 tsp. | 6 tsp. | 7 tsp. | 8 tsp. | 8 tsp. |

### FOOD CHOICES

Breakfast: _____  Lunch: _____

Dinner: _____  Snacks: _____

**Day One**

| Group | Fruits | Vegetables | Grains | Meat & Beans | Milk | Oils |
|-------|--------|------------|--------|--------------|------|------|
| Goal Amount | | | | | | |
| Estimate Your Total | | | | | | |
| Increase ⇧ or Decrease ⇩ ? | | | | | | |

PHYSICAL ACTIVITY

Description: _____

Steps/Miles/Minutes: _____

SPIRITUAL ACTIVITY

Description: _____

_____

### FOOD CHOICES

Breakfast: _____  Lunch: _____

Dinner: _____  Snacks: _____

**Day Two**

| Group | Fruits | Vegetables | Grains | Meat & Beans | Milk | Oils |
|-------|--------|------------|--------|--------------|------|------|
| Goal Amount | | | | | | |
| Estimate Your Total | | | | | | |
| Increase ⇧ or Decrease ⇩ ? | | | | | | |

PHYSICAL ACTIVITY

Description: _____

Steps/Miles/Minutes: _____

SPIRITUAL ACTIVITY

Description: _____

_____

### FOOD CHOICES

Breakfast: _____  Lunch: _____

Dinner: _____  Snacks: _____

**Day Three**

| Group | Fruits | Vegetables | Grains | Meat & Beans | Milk | Oils |
|-------|--------|------------|--------|--------------|------|------|
| Goal Amount | | | | | | |
| Estimate Your Total | | | | | | |
| Increase ⇧ or Decrease ⇩ ? | | | | | | |

PHYSICAL ACTIVITY

Description: _____

Steps/Miles/Minutes: _____

SPIRITUAL ACTIVITY

Description: _____

_____

## Day Four

### FOOD CHOICES

Breakfast: _____ Lunch: _____

Dinner: _____ Snacks: _____

| Group | Fruits | Vegetables | Grains | Meat & Beans | Milk | Oils |
|---|---|---|---|---|---|---|
| Goal Amount | | | | | | |
| Estimate Your Total | | | | | | |
| Increase ⇧ or Decrease ⇩ ? | | | | | | |

**PHYSICAL ACTIVITY**

Description: _____

Steps/Miles/Minutes: _____

**SPIRITUAL ACTIVITY**

Description: _____

_____

## Day Five

### FOOD CHOICES

Breakfast: _____ Lunch: _____

Dinner: _____ Snacks: _____

| Group | Fruits | Vegetables | Grains | Meat & Beans | Milk | Oils |
|---|---|---|---|---|---|---|
| Goal Amount | | | | | | |
| Estimate Your Total | | | | | | |
| Increase ⇧ or Decrease ⇩ ? | | | | | | |

**PHYSICAL ACTIVITY**

Description: _____

Steps/Miles/Minutes: _____

**SPIRITUAL ACTIVITY**

Description: _____

_____

## Day Six

### FOOD CHOICES

Breakfast: _____ Lunch: _____

Dinner: _____ Snacks: _____

| Group | Fruits | Vegetables | Grains | Meat & Beans | Milk | Oils |
|---|---|---|---|---|---|---|
| Goal Amount | | | | | | |
| Estimate Your Total | | | | | | |
| Increase ⇧ or Decrease ⇩ ? | | | | | | |

**PHYSICAL ACTIVITY**

Description: _____

Steps/Miles/Minutes: _____

**SPIRITUAL ACTIVITY**

Description: _____

_____

## Day Seven

### FOOD CHOICES

Breakfast: _____ Lunch: _____

Dinner: _____ Snacks: _____

| Group | Fruits | Vegetables | Grains | Meat & Beans | Milk | Oils |
|---|---|---|---|---|---|---|
| Goal Amount | | | | | | |
| Estimate Your Total | | | | | | |
| Increase ⇧ or Decrease ⇩ ? | | | | | | |

**PHYSICAL ACTIVITY**

Description: _____

Steps/Miles/Minutes: _____

**SPIRITUAL ACTIVITY**

Description: _____

_____

# Live It Tracker

Name: _____    My week at a glance: ☐ Great  ☐ So-so  ☐ Not so great

Date: _____ Week #: _____ Calorie Range: _____    My food goal for next week: _____

Activity Level: None, < 30 min/day, 30-60 min/day, 60+ min/day    My activity goal for next week: _____

Scripture Memory Verse: _____

## RECOMMENDED DAILY AMOUNT OF FOOD FROM EACH GROUP

| Group | Daily Calories | | | | | | | |
|-------|------|------|------|------|------|------|------|------|
| | 1300-1400 | 1500-1600 | 1700-1800 | 1900-2000 | 2100-2200 | 2300-2400 | 2500-2600 | 2700-2800 |
| Fruits | 1.5-2 c. | 1.5-2 c. | 1.5-2 c. | 2-2.5 c. | 2-2.5 c. | 2.5-3.5 c. | 3.5-4.5 c. | 3.5-4.5 c. |
| Vegetables | 1.5-2 c. | 2-2.5 c. | 2.5-3 c. | 2.5-3 c. | 3-3.5 c. | 3.5-4.5 c. | 4.5-5 c. | 4.5-5 c. |
| Grains | 5 oz-eq. | 5-6 oz-eq. | 6-7 oz-eq. | 6-7 oz-eq. | 7-8 oz-eq. | 8-9 oz-eq. | 9-10 oz-eq. | 10-11 oz-eq. |
| Meat & Beans | 4 oz-eq. | 5 oz-eq. | 5-5.5 oz-eq. | 5.5-6.5 oz-eq. | 6.5-7 oz-eq. | 7-7.5 oz-eq. | 7-7.5 oz-eq. | 7.5-8 oz-eq. |
| Milk | 2-3 c. | 3 c. | 3 c. | 3 c. | 3 c. | 3 c. | 3 c. | 3 c. |
| Healthy Oils | 4 tsp. | 5 tsp. | 5 tsp. | 6 tsp. | 6 tsp. | 7 tsp. | 8 tsp. | 8 tsp. |

### Day One

**FOOD CHOICES**

Breakfast: _____    Lunch: _____

Dinner: _____    Snacks: _____

| Group | Fruits | Vegetables | Grains | Meat & Beans | Milk | Oils |
|-------|--------|------------|--------|--------------|------|------|
| Goal Amount | | | | | | |
| Estimate Your Total | | | | | | |
| Increase ⬆ or Decrease ⬇ ? | | | | | | |

**PHYSICAL ACTIVITY**    **SPIRITUAL ACTIVITY**

Description: _____    Description: _____

Steps/Miles/Minutes: _____    _____

### Day Two

**FOOD CHOICES**

Breakfast: _____    Lunch: _____

Dinner: _____    Snacks: _____

| Group | Fruits | Vegetables | Grains | Meat & Beans | Milk | Oils |
|-------|--------|------------|--------|--------------|------|------|
| Goal Amount | | | | | | |
| Estimate Your Total | | | | | | |
| Increase ⬆ or Decrease ⬇ ? | | | | | | |

**PHYSICAL ACTIVITY**    **SPIRITUAL ACTIVITY**

Description: _____    Description: _____

Steps/Miles/Minutes: _____    _____

### Day Three

**FOOD CHOICES**

Breakfast: _____    Lunch: _____

Dinner: _____    Snacks: _____

| Group | Fruits | Vegetables | Grains | Meat & Beans | Milk | Oils |
|-------|--------|------------|--------|--------------|------|------|
| Goal Amount | | | | | | |
| Estimate Your Total | | | | | | |
| Increase ⬆ or Decrease ⬇ ? | | | | | | |

**PHYSICAL ACTIVITY**    **SPIRITUAL ACTIVITY**

Description: _____    Description: _____

Steps/Miles/Minutes: _____    _____

## Day Four

FOOD CHOICES

Breakfast: _____  Lunch: _____

Dinner: _____  Snacks: _____

| Group | Fruits | Vegetables | Grains | Meat & Beans | Milk | Oils |
|---|---|---|---|---|---|---|
| Goal Amount | | | | | | |
| Estimate Your Total | | | | | | |
| Increase ⇧ or Decrease ⇩ ? | | | | | | |

PHYSICAL ACTIVITY

Description: _____

Steps/Miles/Minutes: _____

SPIRITUAL ACTIVITY

Description: _____

_____

## Day Five

FOOD CHOICES

Breakfast: _____  Lunch: _____

Dinner: _____  Snacks: _____

| Group | Fruits | Vegetables | Grains | Meat & Beans | Milk | Oils |
|---|---|---|---|---|---|---|
| Goal Amount | | | | | | |
| Estimate Your Total | | | | | | |
| Increase ⇧ or Decrease ⇩ ? | | | | | | |

PHYSICAL ACTIVITY

Description: _____

Steps/Miles/Minutes: _____

SPIRITUAL ACTIVITY

Description: _____

_____

## Day Six

FOOD CHOICES

Breakfast: _____  Lunch: _____

Dinner: _____  Snacks: _____

| Group | Fruits | Vegetables | Grains | Meat & Beans | Milk | Oils |
|---|---|---|---|---|---|---|
| Goal Amount | | | | | | |
| Estimate Your Total | | | | | | |
| Increase ⇧ or Decrease ⇩ ? | | | | | | |

PHYSICAL ACTIVITY

Description: _____

Steps/Miles/Minutes: _____

SPIRITUAL ACTIVITY

Description: _____

_____

## Day Seven

FOOD CHOICES

Breakfast: _____  Lunch: _____

Dinner: _____  Snacks: _____

| Group | Fruits | Vegetables | Grains | Meat & Beans | Milk | Oils |
|---|---|---|---|---|---|---|
| Goal Amount | | | | | | |
| Estimate Your Total | | | | | | |
| Increase ⇧ or Decrease ⇩ ? | | | | | | |

PHYSICAL ACTIVITY

Description: _____

Steps/Miles/Minutes: _____

SPIRITUAL ACTIVITY

Description: _____

_____

# Live It Tracker

Name: _____     My week at a glance: ☐ Great  ☐ So-so  ☐ Not so great

Date: _____ Week #: _____ Calorie Range: _____     My food goal for next week: _____

Activity Level: None, < 30 min/day, 30-60 min/day, 60+ min/day   My activity goal for next week: _____

Scripture Memory Verse: _____

## RECOMMENDED DAILY AMOUNT OF FOOD FROM EACH GROUP

| Group | Daily Calories | | | | | | | |
|---|---|---|---|---|---|---|---|---|
| | 1300-1400 | 1500-1600 | 1700-1800 | 1900-2000 | 2100-2200 | 2300-2400 | 2500-2600 | 2700-2800 |
| Fruits | 1.5-2 c. | 1.5-2 c. | 1.5-2 c. | 2-2.5 c. | 2-2.5 c. | 2.5-3.5 c. | 3.5-4.5 c. | 3.5-4.5 c. |
| Vegetables | 1.5-2 c. | 2-2.5 c. | 2.5-3 c. | 2.5-3 c. | 3-3.5 c. | 3.5-4.5 c. | 4.5-5 c. | 4.5-5 c. |
| Grains | 5 oz-eq. | 5-6 oz-eq. | 6-7 oz-eq. | 6-7 oz-eq. | 7-8 oz-eq. | 8-9 oz-eq. | 9-10 oz-eq. | 10-11 oz-eq. |
| Meat & Beans | 4 oz-eq. | 5 oz-eq. | 5-5.5 oz-eq. | 5.5-6.5 oz-eq. | 6.5-7 oz-eq. | 7-7.5 oz-eq. | 7-7.5 oz-eq. | 7.5-8 oz-eq. |
| Milk | 2-3 c. | 3 c. | 3 c. | 3 c. | 3 c. | 3 c. | 3 c. | 3 c. |
| Healthy Oils | 4 tsp. | 5 tsp. | 5 tsp. | 6 tsp. | 6 tsp. | 7 tsp. | 8 tsp. | 8 tsp. |

### Day One

**FOOD CHOICES**

Breakfast: _____     Lunch: _____

Dinner: _____     Snacks: _____

| Group | Fruits | Vegetables | Grains | Meat & Beans | Milk | Oils |
|---|---|---|---|---|---|---|
| Goal Amount | | | | | | |
| Estimate Your Total | | | | | | |
| Increase ⇧ or Decrease ⇩ ? | | | | | | |

**PHYSICAL ACTIVITY**

Description: _____

Steps/Miles/Minutes: _____

**SPIRITUAL ACTIVITY**

Description: _____

_____

### Day Two

**FOOD CHOICES**

Breakfast: _____     Lunch: _____

Dinner: _____     Snacks: _____

| Group | Fruits | Vegetables | Grains | Meat & Beans | Milk | Oils |
|---|---|---|---|---|---|---|
| Goal Amount | | | | | | |
| Estimate Your Total | | | | | | |
| Increase ⇧ or Decrease ⇩ ? | | | | | | |

**PHYSICAL ACTIVITY**

Description: _____

Steps/Miles/Minutes: _____

**SPIRITUAL ACTIVITY**

Description: _____

_____

### Day Three

**FOOD CHOICES**

Breakfast: _____     Lunch: _____

Dinner: _____     Snacks: _____

| Group | Fruits | Vegetables | Grains | Meat & Beans | Milk | Oils |
|---|---|---|---|---|---|---|
| Goal Amount | | | | | | |
| Estimate Your Total | | | | | | |
| Increase ⇧ or Decrease ⇩ ? | | | | | | |

**PHYSICAL ACTIVITY**

Description: _____

Steps/Miles/Minutes: _____

**SPIRITUAL ACTIVITY**

Description: _____

_____

## Day Four

### FOOD CHOICES

Breakfast: _____ Lunch: _____

Dinner: _____ Snacks: _____

| Group | Fruits | Vegetables | Grains | Meat & Beans | Milk | Oils |
|---|---|---|---|---|---|---|
| Goal Amount | | | | | | |
| Estimate Your Total | | | | | | |
| Increase ⇧ or Decrease ⇩ ? | | | | | | |

### PHYSICAL ACTIVITY

Description: _____

Steps/Miles/Minutes: _____

### SPIRITUAL ACTIVITY

Description: _____

_____

## Day Five

### FOOD CHOICES

Breakfast: _____ Lunch: _____

Dinner: _____ Snacks: _____

| Group | Fruits | Vegetables | Grains | Meat & Beans | Milk | Oils |
|---|---|---|---|---|---|---|
| Goal Amount | | | | | | |
| Estimate Your Total | | | | | | |
| Increase ⇧ or Decrease ⇩ ? | | | | | | |

### PHYSICAL ACTIVITY

Description: _____

Steps/Miles/Minutes: _____

### SPIRITUAL ACTIVITY

Description: _____

_____

## Day Six

### FOOD CHOICES

Breakfast: _____ Lunch: _____

Dinner: _____ Snacks: _____

| Group | Fruits | Vegetables | Grains | Meat & Beans | Milk | Oils |
|---|---|---|---|---|---|---|
| Goal Amount | | | | | | |
| Estimate Your Total | | | | | | |
| Increase ⇧ or Decrease ⇩ ? | | | | | | |

### PHYSICAL ACTIVITY

Description: _____

Steps/Miles/Minutes: _____

### SPIRITUAL ACTIVITY

Description: _____

_____

## Day Seven

### FOOD CHOICES

Breakfast: _____ Lunch: _____

Dinner: _____ Snacks: _____

| Group | Fruits | Vegetables | Grains | Meat & Beans | Milk | Oils |
|---|---|---|---|---|---|---|
| Goal Amount | | | | | | |
| Estimate Your Total | | | | | | |
| Increase ⇧ or Decrease ⇩ ? | | | | | | |

### PHYSICAL ACTIVITY

Description: _____

Steps/Miles/Minutes: _____

### SPIRITUAL ACTIVITY

Description: _____

_____

# Live It Tracker

Name: _____    My week at a glance:  ☐ Great  ☐ So-so  ☐ Not so great

Date: _____ Week #: _____ Calorie Range: _____  My food goal for next week: _____

Activity Level: None, < 30 min/day, 30-60 min/day, 60+ min/day   My activity goal for next week: _____

Scripture Memory Verse: _____

## RECOMMENDED DAILY AMOUNT OF FOOD FROM EACH GROUP

| Group | Daily Calories | | | | | | | |
|---|---|---|---|---|---|---|---|---|
| | 1300-1400 | 1500-1600 | 1700-1800 | 1900-2000 | 2100-2200 | 2300-2400 | 2500-2600 | 2700-2800 |
| Fruits | 1.5-2 c. | 1.5-2 c. | 1.5-2 c. | 2-2.5 c. | 2-2.5 c. | 2.5-3.5 c. | 3.5-4.5 c. | 3.5-4.5 c. |
| Vegetables | 1.5-2 c. | 2-2.5 c. | 2.5-3 c. | 2.5-3 c. | 3-3.5 c. | 3.5-4.5 c. | 4.5-5 c. | 4.5-5 c. |
| Grains | 5 oz-eq. | 5-6 oz-eq. | 6-7 oz-eq. | 6-7 oz-eq. | 7-8 oz-eq. | 8-9 oz-eq. | 9-10 oz-eq. | 10-11 oz-eq. |
| Meat & Beans | 4 oz-eq. | 5 oz-eq. | 5-5.5 oz-eq. | 5.5-6.5 oz-eq. | 6.5-7 oz-eq. | 7-7.5 oz-eq. | 7-7.5 oz-eq. | 7.5-8 oz-eq. |
| Milk | 2-3 c. | 3 c. | 3 c. | 3 c. | 3 c. | 3 c. | 3 c. | 3 c. |
| Healthy Oils | 4 tsp. | 5 tsp. | 5 tsp. | 6 tsp. | 6 tsp. | 7 tsp. | 8 tsp. | 8 tsp. |

### Day One

FOOD CHOICES

Breakfast: _____    Lunch: _____

Dinner: _____    Snacks: _____

| Group | Fruits | Vegetables | Grains | Meat & Beans | Milk | Oils |
|---|---|---|---|---|---|---|
| Goal Amount | | | | | | |
| Estimate Your Total | | | | | | |
| Increase ⇧ or Decrease ⇩ ? | | | | | | |

PHYSICAL ACTIVITY

Description: _____

Steps/Miles/Minutes: _____

SPIRITUAL ACTIVITY

Description: _____

_____

### Day Two

FOOD CHOICES

Breakfast: _____    Lunch: _____

Dinner: _____    Snacks: _____

| Group | Fruits | Vegetables | Grains | Meat & Beans | Milk | Oils |
|---|---|---|---|---|---|---|
| Goal Amount | | | | | | |
| Estimate Your Total | | | | | | |
| Increase ⇧ or Decrease ⇩ ? | | | | | | |

PHYSICAL ACTIVITY

Description: _____

Steps/Miles/Minutes: _____

SPIRITUAL ACTIVITY

Description: _____

_____

### Day Three

FOOD CHOICES

Breakfast: _____    Lunch: _____

Dinner: _____    Snacks: _____

| Group | Fruits | Vegetables | Grains | Meat & Beans | Milk | Oils |
|---|---|---|---|---|---|---|
| Goal Amount | | | | | | |
| Estimate Your Total | | | | | | |
| Increase ⇧ or Decrease ⇩ ? | | | | | | |

PHYSICAL ACTIVITY

Description: _____

Steps/Miles/Minutes: _____

SPIRITUAL ACTIVITY

Description: _____

_____

## FOOD CHOICES

**Day Four**

Breakfast: _____ Lunch: _____

Dinner: _____ Snacks: _____

| Group | Fruits | Vegetables | Grains | Meat & Beans | Milk | Oils |
|---|---|---|---|---|---|---|
| Goal Amount | | | | | | |
| Estimate Your Total | | | | | | |
| Increase ⇧ or Decrease ⇩ ? | | | | | | |

### PHYSICAL ACTIVITY

Description: _____

Steps/Miles/Minutes: _____

### SPIRITUAL ACTIVITY

Description: _____

_____

---

## FOOD CHOICES

**Day Five**

Breakfast: _____ Lunch: _____

Dinner: _____ Snacks: _____

| Group | Fruits | Vegetables | Grains | Meat & Beans | Milk | Oils |
|---|---|---|---|---|---|---|
| Goal Amount | | | | | | |
| Estimate Your Total | | | | | | |
| Increase ⇧ or Decrease ⇩ ? | | | | | | |

### PHYSICAL ACTIVITY

Description: _____

Steps/Miles/Minutes: _____

### SPIRITUAL ACTIVITY

Description: _____

_____

---

## FOOD CHOICES

**Day Six**

Breakfast: _____ Lunch: _____

Dinner: _____ Snacks: _____

| Group | Fruits | Vegetables | Grains | Meat & Beans | Milk | Oils |
|---|---|---|---|---|---|---|
| Goal Amount | | | | | | |
| Estimate Your Total | | | | | | |
| Increase ⇧ or Decrease ⇩ ? | | | | | | |

### PHYSICAL ACTIVITY

Description: _____

Steps/Miles/Minutes: _____

### SPIRITUAL ACTIVITY

Description: _____

_____

---

## FOOD CHOICES

**Day Seven**

Breakfast: _____ Lunch: _____

Dinner: _____ Snacks: _____

| Group | Fruits | Vegetables | Grains | Meat & Beans | Milk | Oils |
|---|---|---|---|---|---|---|
| Goal Amount | | | | | | |
| Estimate Your Total | | | | | | |
| Increase ⇧ or Decrease ⇩ ? | | | | | | |

### PHYSICAL ACTIVITY

Description: _____

Steps/Miles/Minutes: _____

### SPIRITUAL ACTIVITY

Description: _____

_____

# Live It Tracker

Name: _____  My week at a glance: ❑ Great  ❑ So-so  ❑ Not so great

Date: _____ Week #: _____ Calorie Range: _____  My food goal for next week: _____

Activity Level: None, < 30 min/day, 30-60 min/day, 60+ min/day  My activity goal for next week: _____

Scripture Memory Verse: _____

## RECOMMENDED DAILY AMOUNT OF FOOD FROM EACH GROUP

| Group | Daily Calories | | | | | | | |
|---|---|---|---|---|---|---|---|---|
| | 1300-1400 | 1500-1600 | 1700-1800 | 1900-2000 | 2100-2200 | 2300-2400 | 2500-2600 | 2700-2800 |
| Fruits | 1.5-2 c. | 1.5-2 c. | 1.5-2 c. | 2-2.5 c. | 2-2.5 c. | 2.5-3.5 c. | 3.5-4.5 c. | 3.5-4.5 c. |
| Vegetables | 1.5-2 c. | 2-2.5 c. | 2.5-3 c. | 2.5-3 c. | 3-3.5 c. | 3.5-4.5 c. | 4.5-5 c. | 4.5-5 c. |
| Grains | 5 oz-eq. | 5-6 oz-eq. | 6-7 oz-eq. | 6-7 oz-eq. | 7-8 oz-eq. | 8-9 oz-eq. | 9-10 oz-eq. | 10-11 oz-eq. |
| Meat & Beans | 4 oz-eq. | 5 oz-eq. | 5-5.5 oz-eq. | 5.5-6.5 oz-eq. | 6.5-7 oz-eq. | 7-7.5 oz-eq. | 7-7.5 oz-eq. | 7.5-8 oz-eq. |
| Milk | 2-3 c. | 3 c. | 3 c. | 3 c. | 3 c. | 3 c. | 3 c. | 3 c. |
| Healthy Oils | 4 tsp. | 5 tsp. | 5 tsp. | 6 tsp. | 6 tsp. | 7 tsp. | 8 tsp. | 8 tsp. |

### Day One

**FOOD CHOICES**

Breakfast: _____  Lunch: _____

Dinner: _____  Snacks: _____

| Group | Fruits | Vegetables | Grains | Meat & Beans | Milk | Oils |
|---|---|---|---|---|---|---|
| Goal Amount | | | | | | |
| Estimate Your Total | | | | | | |
| Increase ⇧ or Decrease ⇩ ? | | | | | | |

**PHYSICAL ACTIVITY**                     **SPIRITUAL ACTIVITY**

Description: _____  Description: _____

Steps/Miles/Minutes: _____  _____

### Day Two

**FOOD CHOICES**

Breakfast: _____  Lunch: _____

Dinner: _____  Snacks: _____

| Group | Fruits | Vegetables | Grains | Meat & Beans | Milk | Oils |
|---|---|---|---|---|---|---|
| Goal Amount | | | | | | |
| Estimate Your Total | | | | | | |
| Increase ⇧ or Decrease ⇩ ? | | | | | | |

**PHYSICAL ACTIVITY**                     **SPIRITUAL ACTIVITY**

Description: _____  Description: _____

Steps/Miles/Minutes: _____  _____

### Day Three

**FOOD CHOICES**

Breakfast: _____  Lunch: _____

Dinner: _____  Snacks: _____

| Group | Fruits | Vegetables | Grains | Meat & Beans | Milk | Oils |
|---|---|---|---|---|---|---|
| Goal Amount | | | | | | |
| Estimate Your Total | | | | | | |
| Increase ⇧ or Decrease ⇩ ? | | | | | | |

**PHYSICAL ACTIVITY**                     **SPIRITUAL ACTIVITY**

Description: _____  Description: _____

Steps/Miles/Minutes: _____  _____

## Day Four

**FOOD CHOICES**

Breakfast: _____  Lunch: _____

Dinner: _____  Snacks: _____

| Group | Fruits | Vegetables | Grains | Meat & Beans | Milk | Oils |
|---|---|---|---|---|---|---|
| Goal Amount | | | | | | |
| Estimate Your Total | | | | | | |
| Increase ⇧ or Decrease ⇩ ? | | | | | | |

**PHYSICAL ACTIVITY**

Description: _____

Steps/Miles/Minutes: _____

**SPIRITUAL ACTIVITY**

Description: _____

_____

## Day Five

**FOOD CHOICES**

Breakfast: _____  Lunch: _____

Dinner: _____  Snacks: _____

| Group | Fruits | Vegetables | Grains | Meat & Beans | Milk | Oils |
|---|---|---|---|---|---|---|
| Goal Amount | | | | | | |
| Estimate Your Total | | | | | | |
| Increase ⇧ or Decrease ⇩ ? | | | | | | |

**PHYSICAL ACTIVITY**

Description: _____

Steps/Miles/Minutes: _____

**SPIRITUAL ACTIVITY**

Description: _____

_____

## Day Six

**FOOD CHOICES**

Breakfast: _____  Lunch: _____

Dinner: _____  Snacks: _____

| Group | Fruits | Vegetables | Grains | Meat & Beans | Milk | Oils |
|---|---|---|---|---|---|---|
| Goal Amount | | | | | | |
| Estimate Your Total | | | | | | |
| Increase ⇧ or Decrease ⇩ ? | | | | | | |

**PHYSICAL ACTIVITY**

Description: _____

Steps/Miles/Minutes: _____

**SPIRITUAL ACTIVITY**

Description: _____

_____

## Day Seven

**FOOD CHOICES**

Breakfast: _____  Lunch: _____

Dinner: _____  Snacks: _____

| Group | Fruits | Vegetables | Grains | Meat & Beans | Milk | Oils |
|---|---|---|---|---|---|---|
| Goal Amount | | | | | | |
| Estimate Your Total | | | | | | |
| Increase ⇧ or Decrease ⇩ ? | | | | | | |

**PHYSICAL ACTIVITY**

Description: _____

Steps/Miles/Minutes: _____

**SPIRITUAL ACTIVITY**

Description: _____

_____

# let's count our miles!

## Join the 100-Mile Club this Session

Can't walk that mile yet? Don't be discouraged! There are exercises you can do to strengthen your body and burn those extra calories. Keep a record on your Live It Tracker of the number of minutes you do these common physical activities and then convert those minutes to miles following the chart below. Report your miles to your 100-Mile Club representative when you first arrive each week. Remember, you are not competing with anyone else . . . just yourself. Your job is to strive to reach 100 miles before the last meeting in this session. You can do it—just keep on moving!

### Walking

| | |
|---|---|
| slowly, 2 mph | 30 min. = 156 cal. = 1 mile |
| moderately, 3 mph | 20 min. = 156 cal. = 1 mile |
| very briskly, 4 mph | 15 min. = 156 cal. = 1 mile |
| speed walking | 10 min. = 156 cal. = 1 mile |
| up stairs | 13 min. = 159 cal. = 1 mile |

### Running/Jogging
10 min. = 156 cal. = 1 mile

### Cycling Outdoors

| | |
|---|---|
| slowly, < 10 mph | 20 min. = 156 cal. = 1 mile |
| light effort, 10-12 mph | 12 min. = 156 cal. = 1 mile |
| moderate effort, 12-14 mph | 10 min. = 156 cal. = 1 mile |
| vigorous effort, 14-16 mph | 7.5 min. = 156 cal. = 1 mile |
| very fast, 16-19 mph | 6.5 min. = 152 cal. = 1 mile |

### Sports Activities

| | |
|---|---|
| Playing tennis (singles) | 10 min. = 156 cal. = 1 mile |
| Swimming | |
|   light to moderate effort | 11 min. = 152 cal. = 1 mile |
|   fast, vigorous effort | 7.5 min. = 156 cal. = 1 mile |
| Softball | 15 min. = 156 cal. = 1 mile |
| Golf | 20 min. = 156 cal. = 1 mile |
| Rollerblading | 6.5 min. = 152 cal. = 1 mile |
| Ice skating | 11 min. = 152 cal. = 1 mile |
| Jumping rope | 7.5 min. = 156 cal. = 1 mile |

| Basketball | 12 min. = 156 cal. = 1 mile |
| Soccer (casual) | 15 min. = 159 cal. = 1 mile |

### Around the House

| Mowing grass | 22 min. = 156 cal. = 1 mile |
| Mopping, sweeping, vacuuming | 19.5 min. = 155 cal. = 1 mile |
| Cooking | 40 min. =160 cal. = 1 mile |
| Gardening | 19 min. = 156 cal. = 1 mile |
| Housework (general) | 35 min. = 156 cal. = 1 mile |
| Ironing | 45 min. = 153 cal. = 1 mile |
| Raking leaves | 25 min. = 150 cal. = 1 mile |
| Washing car | 23 min. = 156 cal. = 1 mile |
| Washing dishes | 45 min. = 153 cal. = 1 mile |

### At the Gym

| Stair machine | 8.5 min. = 155 cal. = 1 mile |
| Stationary bike | |
|   slowly, 10 mph | 30 min. = 156 cal. = 1 mile |
|   moderately, 10-13 mph | 15 min. = 156 cal. = 1 mile |
|   vigorously, 13-16 mph | 7.5 min. = 156 cal. = 1 mile |
|   briskly, 16-19 mph | 6.5 min. = 156 cal. = 1 mile |
| Elliptical trainer | 12 min. = 156 cal. = 1 mile |
| Weight machines (used vigorously) | 13 min. = 152 cal. = 1 mile |
| Aerobics | |
|   low impact | 15 min. = 156 cal. = 1 mile |
|   high impact | 12 min. = 156 cal. = 1 mile |
|   water | 20 min. = 156 cal. = 1 mile |
| Pilates | 15 min. = 156 cal. = 1 mile |
| Raquetball (casual) | 15 min. = 159 cal. = 1 mile |
| Stretching exercises | 25 min. = 150 cal. = 1 mile |
| Weight lifting | 30 min. = 156 cal. = 1 mile |
| (would also work for weight machines used moderately or gently) | |

### Family Leisure

| Playing piano | 37 min. = 155 cal. = 1 mile |
| Jumping rope | 10 min. = 152 cal. = 1 mile |
| Skating (moderate) | 20 min. = 152 cal. = 1 mile |
| Swimming | |
|   moderate | 17 min. = 156 cal. = 1 mile |
|   vigorous | 10 min. = 148 cal. = 1 mile |
| Table tennis | 25 min. = 150 cal. = 1 mile |
| Walk/run/play with kids | 25 min. = 150 cal. = 1 mile |

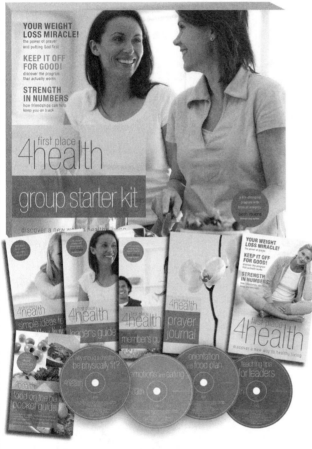
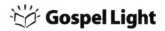

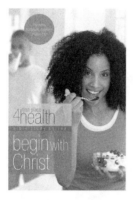
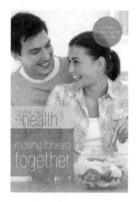
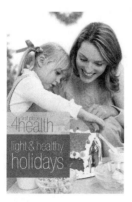
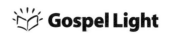

*I press on toward the goal to win the prize for which God has called me heavenward in Christ Jesus.*

Week 3: Stepping Forward in Faith

*By faith Abraham, when called to go to a place he would later receive as his inheritance, obeyed and went, even though he did not know where he was going.*

# Moving Forward Together

*Moving Forward Together*
Scripture Memory Verses:

| | |
|---|---|
| PHILIPPIANS 3:14 | 1 CORINTHIANS 9:24 |
| HEBREWS 11:8 | 1 PETER 5:4 |
| MARK 4:19 | HEBREWS 12:1 |
| COLOSSIANS 3:14 | HEBREWS 12:2 |
| 1 TIMOTHY 6:11 | HEBREWS 12:15 |

PHILIPPIANS 3:14

HEBREWS 11:8

## HOW TO USE THESE CARDS:

Separate cards from the Bible study book. These cards are designed to be used when exercising. To do this, you may want to punch a hole in the upper left corner of the cards and place on a ring. When you have finished memorizing all the verses from one study, add the new Bible study cards to the ring and continue practicing the old verses while learning the new ones. Cards may be placed anywhere you will see them regularly—on the dashboard of your car, on a mirror, on a desk. After you have memorized the verse, begin using the reverse side of the card so the reference is connected to the verse. This is a great way to practice the verses you have already learned.

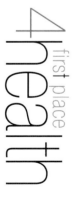

first place
4health

discover a new way to healthy living

Week 6: Pursuit Presses On

*But you, man of God,
flee from all this, and pursue
righteousness, godliness, faith,
love, endurance and gentleness.*

Week 7: All Who Run Can Win

*Do you not know that in a race
all the runners run, but only one
gets the prize? Run in such a
way as to get the prize.*

Week 4: Receptive to the Word

*But the worries of this life,
the deceitfulness of wealth and the
desires for other things come in and
choke the word, making it unfruitful.*

Week 5: Over It All

*And over all these virtues put
on love, which binds them all
together in perfect unity.*

1 TIMOTHY 6:11

MARK 4:19

1 CORINTHIANS 9:24

COLOSSIANS 3:14

Week 10: Focused on the Prize

*Let us fix our eyes on Jesus, the author and perfecter of our faith, who for the joy set before him endured the cross, scorning its shame, and sat down at the right hand of the throne of God.*

Week 11: Binding It All Together

*See to it that no one misses the grace of God and that no bitter root grows up to cause trouble and defile many.*

Week 8: True Glory

*When the Chief Shepherd appears, you will receive the crown of glory that will never fade away.*

Week 9: Breaking Free

*Therefore, since we are surrounded by such a great cloud of witnesses, let us throw off everything that hinders and the sin that so easily entangles, and let us run with perseverance the race marked out for us.*

HEBREWS 12:2

1 PETER 5:4

HEBREWS 12:15

HEBREWS 12:1